Screening:
Evidence and Practice

Angela E. Raffle
Consultant in Public Health, Bristol Primary Care Trust
and the National Screening Programmes;
Honorary Senior Lecturer, University of Bristol
Department of Social Medicine, UK

J. A. Muir Gray
Programmes Director, UK National Screening
Commitee 1996–2007;
Director of the NHS National Knowledge Service

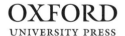

OXFORD
UNIVERSITY PRESS

OXFORD
UNIVERSITY PRESS

Great Clarendon Street, Oxford OX2 6DP

Oxford University Press is a department of the University of Oxford.
It furthers the University's objective of excellence in research, scholarship,
and education by publishing worldwide in

Oxford New York

Auckland Cape Town Dar es Salaam Hong Kong Karachi
Kuala Lumpur Madrid Melbourne Mexico City Nairobi
New Delhi Shanghai Taipei Toronto

With offices in

Argentina Austria Brazil Chile Czech Republic France Greece
Guatemala Hungary Italy Japan Poland Portugal Singapore
South Korea Switzerland Thailand Turkey Ukraine Vietnam

Oxford is a registered trade mark of Oxford University Press
in the UK and in certain other countries

Published in the United States
by Oxford University Press Inc., New York

A catalogue record for this title is available from the British Library

Library of Congress Cataloging in Publication Data
Raffle, Angela E.
    Screening : evidence and practice / Angela E. Raffle, J. A. Muir Gray.
        p. ; cm.
    Includes bibliographical references.
    ISBN 978-0-19-921449-5 (alk. paper)
    1. Medical screening. I. Gray, J. A. Muir (John Armstrong Muir) II. Title.
    [DNLM: 1. Mass screening -- organization & administration. 2. Health Policy.
    3. Mass Screening -- ethics. WA 245 R138s 2007]
    RA427. 5. R34 2007
    362.17'7 -- dc22
                                                                    2007012845

Typeset by Cepha Imaging Private Ltd., Bangalore, India
Printed in Great Britain
on acid-free paper by
Biddles Ltd., King's Lynn, Norfolk

ISBN 978–0–19–921449–5

10 9 8 7 6 5 4 3 2

Contents

Foreword

It is just over 150 years since the concept of identifying the future health risks of individuals surfaced. Today, it would not seem remarkable to the public that individuals can be tested for the potential to develop disease. Whilst many have benefited from the multitude of screening programmes now on offer in the UK, developing these and ensuring that they reach the highest standard has not been without difficulty.

At the heart of this debate is the question best elucidated by Wilson and Junger in 1968 - what should the aims of a screening programme be? Their careful assessment and development of criteria has helped shape the evolution of screening, particularly in the UK. Initial programmes were ad hoc and often failed to fully meet these standards. The development of the National Screening Committee has brought academic rigour and authority to this complex area. The measured direction of this group has guided the introduction of important new initiatives, such as the colorectal cancer and neonatal sickle cell programmes.

The challenges of the past are not ended. The ever-increasing technological and biological wizardry of medicine raises expectations and further stretches clinicians. These challenges are as true for screening. The public health and research communities are responding, and doing so admirably; the UK Collaborative Trial of Ovarian Cancer (UKCTOCS) as cited in this book, is an example of how difficult questions may be researched, if collaboration is sought and rigorous research standards applied.

This book captures the challenges and lays down the gauntlet for the future. But more than this, the book gives the next generation of managers, public health doctors, clinicians and patients the understanding to meet these challenges. By marking the important contribution that screening can and has made, and charting the development of this new and exciting field of medicine, the book presents the power and the potential dangers of screening in a balanced and approachable manner.

Few developments have the potential to minimise suffering to the extent that quality screening can. This book is a timely and substantive reminder of why we screen, and the dangers of doing so. By examining the detailed processes that lead to successful screening programmes at a national and local level, elucidating the complexities of both initiating and perpetuating high quality programmes, the authors will help to ensure that the United Kingdom continues to provide only the best possible screening programmes.

This book manages to explain complex and challenging epidemiological and statistical concepts through thoughtful case examples, clear tutorials, and self-assessment. Whilst gently guiding the novice into this fascinating and difficult area, this unique book further manages to add to the knowledge base of more seasoned health professionals by the in-depth coverage of the subject matter and the detailed analysis of the failures and successes of the past, both within the UK and further afield.

I commend the authors for tackling this topic and by doing so with both breadth and clarity. I am sure that this book will become a valuable resource for the caretakers of screening programmes of the next 150 years.

SIR LIAM DONALDSON

CHIEF MEDICAL OFFICER

DEPARTMENT OF HEALTH

Preface

All screening programmes do harm. Some do good as well and, of these, some do more good than harm at reasonable cost. It is the responsibility of policy makers, public health practitioners, managers and the clinicians involved in screening to ensure that only programmes that do more good than harm at reasonable cost are implemented and, when they are implemented, that they are managed in such a way as to achieve a level of quality which will ensure that the balance of good and harm demonstrated in research is reproduced in the ordinary service setting. Unfortunately, many screening services either have been introduced on the basis of inadequate evidence that they do more good than harm at reasonable cost or, if introduced on good evidence, are managed so badly that the efficacy demonstrated in research is not translated into effectiveness in practice. This results in a waste of resources and in harm to those individuals who accept the offer of screening.

For 20 years we have been involved in policy making, and in subsequent implementation, and management of screening programmes offered to the populations for which we have been responsible. We have also inherited screening programmes from the past that were introduced either without an adequate evidence base or without an adequate management system. This has given us good experience of working our way out of the mess we inherited, in order to achieve a screening programme that does more good than harm at reasonable cost.

During this time, we have had the pleasure of working with many public health practitioners in training, mostly from the UK, but also from a number of other countries, and the teaching material that we have developed is brought together here into this book.

This is a 'how to' book, focusing on the steps that professionals need to take, both directly and in consultation with the population they serve, either to improve the programmes inherited or to ensure that new programmes are based on sound evidence and then implemented in a way that will ensure that benefits demonstrated in research are reproduced in practice. The public health practitioner responsible for screening at a national level usually has to ensure that at least a hundred times as many workers are identified, trained, motivated and informed as were required for the original study on which the policy decision was based.

We have also tried to cover the ethical issues involved in screening because we have found these to be of central importance in our discussions with colleagues, the public and the media. Screening has one important distinction from clinical practice, namely that some of the people who suffer the side effects and harms, inherent in all medical technology, do not have the disease for which screening was initiated and are therefore harmed without any possibility of benefit. When you treat someone who comes to you with an illness, the patient being treated has at least a possibility of benefit as well as a risk of harm.

This book is dedicated to all those we have worked with to improve screening in the UK.

J. A. Muir Gray, CBE, DSc, MD, FRCP, FRCPSGlas, FCILIP
Programmes Director, National Screening Committee

Angela E. Raffle, BSc(Hons), MB ChB, FFPHM
Consultant to the National Screening Programmes

Endorsements

A readable, yet encyclopedic guide to screening: its history, its key design elements, its implementation and its policy challenges. Using case studies and simple figures Raffle and Gray illustrate the fundamental balance involved: many must be tested, so that a few might benefit—while others will invariably be overdiagnosed and treated needlessly. I was intrigued, in particular, by their delineation of two barriers to balanced discussions of screening: firstly, the reassurance illusion—those with a normal screening exam feel good, even though their risk has changed little and secondly, the popularity paradox—the more overdiagnosis a screening program causes, the more popular it is—as more and more participants believe they owe it their life. A must read for clinicians, managers, and policymakers who would like to assist Raffle and Gray in achieving their goal: 'to sort out the mess'.

H. Gilbert Welch
VA Outcomes Group
USA

Intuitively, screening seems to make sense. One would expect that early detection improves health outcomes. However, as Raffle and Gray compellingly show, this often is not the case. Evidence shows that screening for some conditions carries no benefit. And where screening has potential for good, the benefits may be eroded by harms or by poor formulation or implementation of screening policies.

In their marvelous book, Raffle and Gray shine a light that reflects the multifaceted face of screening. They deal with evaluating its benefits and harms; ensuring that worthwhile screening is implemented in a way that realizes its potential; and managing the process of decision-making between public health practitioners, clinicians and the public they serve. The concepts in this book, so clearly explained and illustrated, are strongly based on evidence and the authors' experience and wisdom in using evidence for public health decision-making. *Screening: Evidence and Practice* is destined to be an important read for public health practitioners, clinicians and medical students alike.

Professor Les Irwig
Screening and Test Evaluation Program
School of Public Health
Faculty of Medicine
University of Sydney
AUSTRALIA

The more interested you are in new technologies for health screening, the more you need to read this book. The pathobiological, methodological and logistical aspects of screening for chronic disease seem ever changing, and as technology changes too we seem always to be aiming at moving targets. By reading this book you will gain insights from the historical and cultural contexts in which screening activities usually develop. You will then understand the unstoppable nature of screening, and the obligation to seek for research-based and controlled optimum clinical practice for early detection in high-risk persons. You will also learn that sound screening practice has to be built on the strong foundation of realistic communication with the population at risk.

Professor Jan Willem Coebergh
Professor of Cancer Surveillance at the Erasmus
Medical Centre Rotterdam
Editor of the Epidemiology and Prevention
section of the European Journal of Cancer

Acknowledgements

We would like to thank the following people, all of whom have helped in some way towards this book: Ike Anya, Liz Aram, Alex Barratt, Kay Chamberlain, Jan Willem Coebergh, Adrian Davis, Ann Dixon-Brown, Rachel Foley, Linda Garvican, Winifred Gray, Anne Green, Walter Holland, Les Irwig, Lindsay Kimm, Ruth Kipping, George Knox, Steve Laitner, Rosemary Lees, Judith Maxwell, Liz Midgley, John Murdoch, Jason Ovens, Mike Owen, Nicola Pearce Smith, David Pittaway, Monica Raffle, Julia Rowley, Ann Southwell, Allison Streetly, Heather Sharp, Yoshitaka Tsubono, Gilbert Welch, William Warin, and our anonymous reviewers.

Chapter 1

How screening started

The aim of the chapter

The aim of this chapter is to give knowledge and insight into how health screening began, how the aims of screening have changed during the twentieth century, how the requirement for evidence and organization influenced matters and how challenges in the future will give rise to continuing change. The evolution of screening has followed different courses in different parts of the world, shaped by medical, cultural, commercial and political factors. A full worldwide overview is beyond the scope of this book. We have focused on events in the UK, and in the USA, for which we have relied heavily upon Paul Han's excellent history (Han 1997).

Pre-modern screening

> The ranchman has his annual round-up, the merchant his yearly account of stock and balancing of books; the machinist gives his engine a thorough going-over at regular intervals; every military organisation has its reviews and inspections; every government its budgets.
>
> George Gould (1900)

Early recommendations

In 1861, Dr Horace Dobell, an eminent physician practising at London's Royal Hospital for Chest Diseases, gave a series of lectures culminating in the recommendation that physicians should perform periodic checks on everyone, irrespective of whether they were seeking medical help (Dobell 1861).

> There should be instituted, as a custom, a system of periodical examination, to which all persons should submit themselves, and to which they should submit their children. The examination should be reported in writing; and,

> after due consideration, such advice must be given as careful judgement
> may dictate, for the future conduct, pursuits and habits of the patient. ...;
> such a system of examination and advice as I propose, if properly carried
> out, must strike at the root of these evils, and would at the same time reduce
> the miserable over-crowding of the hospital waiting-rooms, and the enor-
> mous expenses incurred for drugs.

Dobell argued quite validly that most deaths were not solely due to the disease named on the death registration. The real culprit, he argued, was a lack of 'vital force' for fighting disease, which in turn arose from three main influences: living conditions; co-existing disease; and the vestiges of pre-existing diseases, primarily anaemia, fatty degeneration and syphilis. He exhorted his audience to embrace the prevention of ill-health 'a duty as much above the management of acute disease as to rule an empire is above fighting a pitched battle', and he proposed that this could be achieved by a system of comprehensive periodical examinations. He believed that the advice physicians would give following these routine examinations would alter living conditions, and co-existing disease and vestiges of disease, and would thereby prevent future disease. Dobell gave little clue as to the precise nature of the advice that would succeed with this massive task, although he did mention beer, cheese, exercise, oxygen, unsuitable working environments and the wearing of flannel clothing.

The idea of routinely examining ordinary people whilst they were still well was, at that time, highly unusual. For the very wealthy, who did not have to share their attending physicians with others, such precautionary checks were probably not unheard of, but as a general concept this was a novel idea. Dobell's ideas were soon echoed in the USA and elsewhere, coupled with a growing interest in the potential scientific value of collecting data from examining healthy subjects. Yet in the UK during the first half of the twentieth century, the idea was largely ignored, and widespread medical examination of healthy adults, with the aim of preventing disease, did not happen. The only sphere in which screening was routine was within child health programmes, which we explain more of later. Army recruits were examined, but this was a longstanding practice, aimed not at improving the subjects' health but at selecting out those who were physically or mentally unsuited to the needs of the military machine.

In some countries, including the USA, the concept of regular and non-specific health examinations for ordinary adults and children, did take a very firm hold, but not immediately.

The rise of the periodic health examination, 1900–1950

Box 1.1 Gould in Atlantic City

In June 1900, eminent physicians from all over the USA, gathered in the splendid resort of Atlantic City, New Jersey, for the fifty-first annual meeting of the American Medical Association. It was at this meeting that Dr George M. Gould, a physician from Philadelphia, gave a paper that helped sow the seed for instigation of the 'annual periodic examination', the practice whereby many Americans have a routine health examination once a year.

The essence of Gould's argument was that ranchers check their cattle, merchants check their stock, accountants check their books, generals check their armies, governments check their budgets, but doctors do not check their patients—and they should. His lengthy paper 'A system of personal biologic examinations the condition of adequate medical and scientific conduct of life' (Gould 1900) was without a single reference, but this was usual in 1900. The motivation for Gould's recommendation of annual health checks was to understand what caused disease and how to prevent it, thus benefiting future generations.

The arguments that Gould put forward were as follows:

- Collection of comprehensive 'morphologic, physiologic and pathogenic' data would yield understanding of 'the evolution of the organism and of its present departures from a normal standard'. This was Gould's primary argument, and he envisaged annual or five yearly collection of all kinds of data on every individual from birth through to death. The record would include post-mortem data, and storage of preserved organs such as the brain and the skull.

Box 1.1 Gould in Atlantic City *(cont.)*

- Vast amounts of data were already being collected but were not being used scientifically. The existing examples Gould gave included life-insurance medicals, school medical examinations, police criminal records, military examinations, gymnasium tests, hospital and patients records, census records and pensioners' medical examinations. His vision was of 'an extended and perfected bureau of vital statistics'.

- Although it would need resources to collect and use data systematically, this would be only a fraction of that 'being squandered on war' 'poured into the pockets of city bosses' or 'spent on comic opera'.

- If physicians succeeded in convincing patients of the necessity and wisdom of repeated examinations, as dentists had successfully done, then physicians would be able to learn how to prevent symptoms before they ever arose, and pathologists would come to understand how diseases are caused.

- Manifest disease, with signs or symptoms, often went unrecognized and untreated for many years because patients did not consult a doctor. Through regular examinations this disease could be properly diagnosed and treated.

In one part of Gould's speech, and no doubt this brought much laughter from his audience, he speculates on some of the directions in which medicine seemed to be travelling. He suggested that advertisements would soon be seen for 'craniotomy for unselfishness; preventive inoculations for threatened breach of promise; heart-valves surgically repaired while you wait; kidneys transplanted immediately following the next electrocution [and] complete maturation of the artificially fertilised ovum in our new twenty-first century incubator'—all this at a time when heart or transplant surgery, and *in vitro* fertilization were far in the future. Gould's recommendations were optimistic and inspired by humanitarian and scientific motives. However, the concept of periodic examinations did not gain immediate popularity with doctors or with the public, and once they did it was not quite for the reasons that Gould foresaw. Paul Han gives us a valuable overview of the unfolding of events in the USA (Han 1997).

The role of life-insurance companies

It was the life-insurance companies, already used to medical examinations as a means of setting premiums, that began to recommend regular examinations for their policyholders. Data collected by these companies demonstrated that mortality rates in those who persisted with regular exams were substantially lower than expected from actuarial calculations. This is not surprising. Those who have the commitment and stability to continue with regular examinations are a highly selected healthy group, and we cover the phenomenon of selection bias in Chapter 4. However, at the time it was easy to assume cause and effect—it was assumed that the examinations must be the cause of the greater length of life, when in fact it was simply that those with longest life expectancy complied best with regular testing.

The insurance companies' approach influenced the content of the examinations as well as the fact that they happened. The companies' aim was financial risk avoidance, and any defect in any test result was regarded as a risk until proven otherwise. Examinations were exhaustive, and almost all healthy people were found to have some defect. This might have prompted questions over whether these 'defects' might be part of the range of normal. Instead it was seen as proof that the examinations were indeed needed.

The role of employers

Employers in the USA quickly followed the insurance companies in adopting routine periodic examinations for their workforces. The aims were partly to enhance welfare for the workers and improve efficiency and productivity, and partly to protect the employer against injury compensation claims under legislation that had been passed in the early 1900s. By screening, the employer could uncover any pre-existing conditions that might otherwise have been claimed for as induced through work.

Periodic examinations for senior company executives became progressively more wide-ranging and thorough. By the 1950s, the famous Greenbrier Clinic was running a 3-day health check for private industry clients, and in Japan top executives were admitted to hospital for 5 days of health checks, known as the Human Dry Dock (Sasamori 1982). Much of the drive came from a genuine pioneering spirit, reflecting a confidence in the ability of technology to solve problems, although undoubtedly the fees that could be charged were also a factor. At the time, the self-evident principle was 'a stitch in time saves nine', and few stopped to consider that they were expending great effort stitching nearly everything, whether it was starting to rip or not.

The part played by the medical profession

Many physicians were initially reluctant to become engaged in routine periodic checks, feeling that it was not worthwhile and not a good use of their time and expertise. In 1922, however, the American Medical Association officially endorsed the practice of the periodic health examination, and co-operated with major public information campaigns to promote uptake. It was most probably professional self-interest that influenced this. Independent physicians were facing the prospect of losing their exclusive relationship with their patients because public health programmes began to usurp the physicians' role. By participating in screening, they preserved their prime position and avoided surrendering the role to public institutions and government. The historian George Rosen describes how the periodic examination became a weapon in the fierce battle fought by private physicians who opposed compulsory health insurance, school health programmes and municipal health programmes (Rosen 1975). By laying claim to the examination and performing it themselves, they could avert government control of healthcare activity.

Routine use of periodic examination in the 1950s

By the 1950s, the annual periodic health examination had now become standard practice, and yielded vast experience of the technical challenges involved (Thorner 1961). There was a huge growth in literature about test performance and screening theory. The 1950s also brought growing use of 'multiphasic' screening, using automated laboratory processes that enabled whole batteries of tests to be run on a single blood sample. This brought down costs, and enabled even more tests to be incorporated. Healthcare provider organizations in the USA began to provide routine periodic health examinations for their plan members, with the San Francisco Kaiser Permanente Health Plan starting the practice in 1951. Kaiser's experience was that the growing public belief in regular checks caused massive demand for appointments and check-ups from plan members, threatening to overwhelm their resources. Kaiser concluded that a regular system of checks was a more efficient way of managing this patient demand than allowing patients to choose for themselves when to come for examinations (Collen 1974).

The implied purpose of screening had changed fundamentally from the vision described by Gould. A venture that began as a quest for scientific knowledge was now being practised as though there was certain benefit to the individual. The very fact that these tests were done and abnormalities were found was sufficient to convince most people of their value.

Routine testing of healthy people had become a firmly established practice, and the implied objective was reduced risk of future ill health. The major forces that had brought the routine examination into USA practice were:

- Scientific and humanitarian desire to uncover truths about disease causation and prevention
- Insurance companies' use of rigorous and repeated testing of policy-holders in order to minimize financial risk for the companies
- Employers' use of tests for employees, to minimize risk of compensation claims and to achieve a productive workforce
- The medical profession's need to provide the testing, whether they felt it worthwhile or not, in order to resist encroachment by municipal and government healthcare schemes
- Direct campaigns that convinced the public of the value of routine testing
- The need for healthcare plan providers to control unfettered demand for check-ups, which meant that they instigated a regular schedule of checks.

So, almost by accident, the public ended up being tested comprehensively and often, with complete certainty that this was in their own interest. Players in the story had each had their own reasons for promoting testing. Definitive evidence that benefit outweighed harm, or that this was the best way of using healthcare resources, had not been a driving force.

We will soon come to the challenges that began in the 1960s, once the medical profession began to raise serious questions about the value of the routine examination. The timing was disastrous, since by this time public enthusiasm for routine examinations had gained hold, and healthcare providers had become commercially dependent on the practice. However, before we get to the challenges, we first need to consider what happened in the UK before 1960.

Screening in the UK 1900–1950

Even though it was a London physician, Dr Horace Dobell (Dobell 1861), who is credited as being one of the earliest advocates of periodic health checks, the practice was ignored in the UK, except for children Strangely enough, the factor that tipped the balance in favour of child health screening may well have been the publication of a best-selling novel.

Box 1.2 *The riddle of the sands,* **and child health screening in the UK**

The health of children in Britain through the nineteenth century was dreadful, and the plight of the nation's poorest children had been recorded regularly since the first Poor Law Commission of 1834 (Smith 1979). The link between poor child health and the poor health of young men attending army recruitment offices for the Boer Wars, first in the 1880s and subsequently in the 1890s, was not a difficult one to make. Successful public health reforms concerning sanitation, drinking water, housing, food and safe burial of the dead had occurred from the 1850s for the benefit of all strata of society, but few health measures were specifically aimed at the poor and needy. In 1903, the publication of Erskine Childer's novel *The riddle of the sands* met with widespread acclaim and alarm. It is a story of two young Englishmen who set out on a sailing holiday along the German North Sea coast, and find themselves involved in an epic spy adventure. Efforts by the German authorities to send them on their way alert them to sinister possibilities, culminating eventually in their discovery of a secret invasion force hidden in specially constructed canals, and their narrow escape back to England with the crucial intelligence (Childers 1903).

> **Box 1.2** *The riddle of the sands,* **and child health screening in the UK** *(cont.)*
>
> Childers had constructed his brilliantly written novel with serious intent. There were divided feelings in the UK about the potential threat of Germany's growing naval and military strength. Kaiser Wilhelm II of Germany was the grandson of the UK monarch Queen Victoria, and aristocratic ties between the countries were strong. The book successfully mobilized public fears concerning the growing power of the Kaiser's empire, and was followed by changes in naval policy and by the establishment of a Parliamentary Inter-Departmental Committee on Physical Degeneration. The aim of the Committee was to do something about child health in order to improve the fitness of young men needed for military recruitment, as proved necessary once the First World War commenced in 1914. In 1904 (Inter-Departmental Committee 1904), the committee recommended a range of measures, including the prohibition of sale of tobacco and cigarettes in sweet shops and other shops frequented by children, but most importantly it recommended a system of regular medical and dental inspection of schoolchildren. The School Medical Service was thereby established, with responsibility for conducting routine inspections on all schoolchildren. This was well ahead of the UK National Health Service which commenced in 1948, again the product of wartime experience.

Apart from some isolated examples of occupational checks, and the routine enquiries made by insurance companies, regular checks on all adults were unheard of in the UK during the first half of the twentieth century. Mass mobile radiography was used in the 1940s and 1950s as part of tuberculosis control programmes, but this was discontinued once disease prevalence fell. The prevailing attitude amongst patients and doctors alike in pre-1950s Britain was that, provided there was nothing wrong with you, it was best to steer clear of unnecessary and potentially meddlesome investigations.

Modern screening

As a whole, the series leaves the impression that total population screening is hard to justify for any condition, save PKU. Selective screening, on the other hand, has a useful place in health care but a great deal of work remains to be done. The first major area for attention is systematic, stringent, and unemotional evaluation of the various screening procedures for introduction. It is essential for unequivocal evidence to be presented before an experimental project is introduced into routine medical practice.

Walter Holland (1974)

The end of the technological dream

Events emerge gradually, and any divisions that we make looking back—between 'pre-modern' and 'modern' screening for example—are of course arbitrary. In 1950s Britain, awareness of screening was just beginning, whilst in the USA the practice was firmly in place. Then came the 1960s, a time of great upheaval. World events outside of medicine were dominated by challenges to the status quo. In 1968 alone there was the Tet Offensive and the Mai Lai massacre in Vietnam; the French student riots that brought the country to a virtual standstill for weeks necessitating the flight of General de Gaulle; violence in Red Lion Square in London when the far-right National Front clashed with opponents; and 5 days of street battles in Chicago at the Democratic Party Convention. Change was in the air and everything traditional was liable to be challenged.

The key events for screening were:

+ Two reports were published, both in 1968. One was from the Nuffield Provincial Hospitals Trust the other from the World Health Organization (Wilson and Jungner 1968). These began the process of questioning some of the accepted beliefs about screening.

+ Two randomized controlled trials were established, one at Kaiser Permanente in 1964 (Friedman *et al.* 1986) the other in South-East London in 1967 (The South-East London Study Group 1977), with the aim of measuring the impact of periodic examination on mortality rates, on general health and on use of health services.

The report of the Nuffield Provincial Hospitals Trust

There was growing concern amongst rigorously minded academics about the sweeping claims for screening that had been made by apparently authoritative bodies, based on no particular evidence. In 1957, for example, the Commission on Chronic Illness in the USA had been happy to recommend a wide range of screening, for diabetes, glaucoma and cancers of the mouth skin, breast, cervix and rectum, based not on research evidence but on statements such as this:

> increasing numbers of physicians and other health personnel have come to the conclusion that screening tests …; can be an effective device in secondary prevention of chronic illness (Commission on Chronic Illness 1957).

The Nuffield Trust therefore set up a Working Party, under the chairmanship of Tom McKeown, Professor of Social Medicine in Birmingham, UK. McKeown subsequently became legendary in public health circles for his work demonstrating that major health improvements in the nineteenth and twentieth centuries owed more to the impact of food, clean water and decent housing than to the impact of modern medical interventions (McKeown 1976).

The Nuffield Trust Working Party published a series of essays (Nuffield Provincial Hospitals Trust 1968) considering the validation required of screening procedures, and assessing 10 existing or proposed screening activities against these validation criteria. The 10 topics were bacteriuria in pregnancy, breast cancer, cervical cancer, deafness in childhood, diabetes mellitus, glaucoma, iron deficiency anaemia, phenylketonuria, pulmonary tuberculosis and rhesus haemolytic disease of the newborn. Their conclusion was that six of the 10 programmes they examined were 'seriously deficient', meaning that it was not possible to say whether or not the screening did more good than harm. Even for the four that did have valid evidence (deafness, phenylketonuria, tuberculosis and rhesus haemolytic disease) the authors found important gaps in the available information. The overall conclusion, summarized in the Preface, was:

> public funds can be, and it seems may already have been, diverted from fields of certain benefit to procedures which are not proved and possibly harmful (Nuffield Provincial Hospitals Trust 1968).

The book made the case for an expert advisory committee, independent of government, to review the evidence in this complex field. The dangers of not having such an arrangement were underlined. First, premature introduction of screening would make it impossible to obtain essential knowledge based on proper research and, secondly, 'public ignorance, or imperfect understanding, of the problems involved, may lead to pressure on government to provide a screening service before a comprehensive assessment of its worth'.

The Nuffield Trust Report raised questions about the efficiency of screening, as well as the effectiveness. Using data about the costs of screening examinations, the report challenged the widespread assumption that screening would inevitably lead to reduced health-care costs. It showed that routine screening consumes a great deal of resources because of the sheer numbers of subjects that need to be tested. If it is effective, and does more good than harm, then this may well be a worthwhile use of resources. If it is ineffective, then it represents a major lost opportunity for using resources in a more beneficial way.

The introductory chapter by McKeown (1968) also made important statements about the ethical difference between screening and routine medical care. When a patient seeks advice for a complaint the ethical duty of the doctor is to do the best that is possible with the knowledge and resources available. With screening, McKeown argued, the ethics are different.

> There is a presumptive undertaking, not merely that abnormality will be identified if it is present, but that those affected will derive benefit from subsequent treatment or care. This commitment is at least implicit, and except for research and the protection of the public health, no one should be expected to submit to the inconvenience of investigation or the anxieties of case-finding without the prospect of medical benefit. The obligation exists even when the patient asks to be screened, for his request is then based on the belief that the procedure is of value, and if it is not it is for medical people to make this known (McKeown 1968).

Wilson and Jungner's report for the World Health Organization

Aware that the practice of multiphasic screening was growing without any clear evidence or principles to underpin it, the World Health Organization secured the expertise of Drs J.M.G. Wilson and G. Jungner to write a report. Max Wilson was a Principal Medical Officer with the Ministry of Health in London who, at the request of the then Chief Medical Officer George Godber, had spent 6 months in the

USA in 1963 studying the subject of screening. Gunnar Jungner was a senior clinical chemist from Sweden with considerable expertise on matters of test performance.

Their 150 page booklet was published as a Public Health Paper for the World Health Organization (Wilson and Jungner 1968). The style is direct, although at times the content is clearly diplomatic and cautious. The booklet discusses:

- The growth of screening
- The assumptions upon which any presumed benefit of early detection depend
- The deceptiveness of screening's apparent simplicity
- The pitfalls and the scope for harm
- The futility of testing without subsequent action
- The lack of knowledge or information concerning the economics of early detection.

They commented specifically on the fact that most variables measured by a screening test have a unimodal, not a bimodal, distribution. In other words, there is no separation between a group that is definitely destined to develop the disease, and those who are not. They highlight the fact that this has major significance for the problem of categorizing people as 'borderline', and they state that for a screening process:

> the terms 'sensitivity' and 'specificity' ...; have theoretically no meaning for a unimodal distribution (Wilson and Jungner 1968, p. 26).

So already they were highlighting the need for screening theory to encompass more than just test performance. What mattered was whole programme performance in relation to the specific adverse outcome, relating either to morbidity or mortality, that screening was aiming to prevent.

Wilson and Jungner reviewed most of the specific conditions for which early detection had been claimed to bring benefit, and found problems with almost all of them. They set out 10 tentative principles, which they called 'guides to planning case finding'. These 10 principles, as they appear in the original 1968 publication, are listed below.

'Guides to planning case-finding' (Wilson and Jungner 1968, pp. 26–27)

1. The condition sought should be an important health problem.
2. There should be an accepted treatment for patients with recognized disease.
3. Facilities for diagnosis and treatment should be available.
4. There should be a recognizable latent or early symptomatic phase.
5. There should be a suitable test or examination.
6. The test should be acceptable to the population.
7. The natural history of the condition, including development from latent to declared disease, should be adequately understood.
8. There should be an agreed policy on whom to treat as patients.
9. The cost of case-finding (including diagnosis and treatment of patients diagnosed) should be economically balanced in relation to possible expenditure on medical care as a whole.
10. Case-finding should be a continuing process and not a 'once and for all' project.

Their 10 principles have had a dominant and lasting impact on the world literature, and have probably been more often cited than any other publication concerning screening. They have been as much misused as used. Wilson and Jungner put these principles forward as a preliminary checklist, with the reasoning going like this—unless all these conditions can be met then it is probably pointless to consider screening, and it is probably premature to invest in research. If they are met, then careful research is needed to measure the balance of benefit and harm, the affordability, and to elucidate the best means of delivering a programme.

The principles led to an oversimplification of a complex set of questions. The checklist approach tended to suggest that there was always a Yes or No answer, forcing people to take sides and adopt entrenched positions. Often the screening in question had already crept into practice anyway, so the principles tended to be used as justification—if the condition is serious, comes on slowly, and there is some sort of a test, then let's start screening, three out of ten isn't bad. Wilson and

Jungner were not in a position to foresee just how difficult it would be to persuade physicians, public and policy makers that screening needed to be based on evidence. To them it was obvious that evidence was needed just as for any other potentially harmful medical intervention. Yet so powerful was the notion that screening must always be the right thing to do, it has taken years to reach general acceptance that evidence of more good than harm at affordable cost must precede widespread introduction. Even once evidence exists, questions about how best to deliver the screening programme were and are still crucially important.

The two randomized controlled trials of periodic health examination

In 1964, Kaiser Permanente enrolled some 10 000 adults aged 35–64 within their health maintenance organization into a randomized controlled trial.

◆ The intervention group was urged to have annual multiphasic examination. The control group had access to multiphasic examinations on request, but subjects in the control group were not urged to take them up.

◆ The mean number of multiphasic checks during the study was 6.8 for intervention group subjects, and 2.8 for controls.

◆ The results at 7 years and at 16 years (Friedman *et al.* 1986) were published. There was no difference in total mortality or in self-reported disability between the intervention group and the control group.

◆ Mortality data for California, estimated to capture 82–92 per cent of all deaths for the study subjects, were analysed for 34 separate causes of death. For three discrete causes the difference between cases and controls was greater than expected by chance using a 95 per cent confidence interval. The 95 per cent confidence test highlights differences that would only be likely to occur by chance one in 20 times. So for 34 different measures, the chance of finding at least one 'significant' difference becomes virtually certain.

◆ The three differences were: deaths attributed to cancer of the colon and rectum were significantly less in the intervention group, with 12 deaths compared with 29; deaths attributed to haematological cancer were higher in the intervention group, with 22 deaths compared with 10; and deaths attributed to suicide were higher in the intervention group, with 25 deaths compared with 11.

◆ The authors concluded that the reduction in colorectal cancer, and a non-significant reduction in disease related to hypertension, were as a result of the health checks, and that the excess of haematological cancers and suicide were not. Whether this is a valid interpretation is open to question, but the results certainly showed no evidence that multiphasic checks enhanced life or well-being.

So, overall, this trial showed that the way forward with screening lay with the evaluation of programmes using specific screening measures aimed at risk reduction for specific illnesses.

In 1967, at the request of the Department of Health, a trial commenced in South East London involving 7000 adults aged 40–64 followed-up for 9 years (South-East London Study Group 1977).

◆ Two comprehensive multiphasic screenings were carried out, involving a detailed health questionnaire, physical examination and a full range of tests including chest X-ray, lung function, electrocardiogram, blood tests and faecal occult blood.

◆ Uptake at the first screen was 73.4 per cent, and at the second was 65.5 per cent. No screening took place in the control group.

◆ Outcome measures included family doctor consultation rates, hospital admissions, certified sickness absence from work, mortality rates and a final health survey of all subjects, in both the intervention and the control groups, 2 years after the second screen.

◆ No significant differences were found between screening and control groups in any of these measures.

◆ The cost of a multiphasic screen for one adult worked out at £12.27 at 1976 prices, which was one-fifth of the charge being made by private screening clinics at that time in the UK.

The authors concluded that 'the use of general practice based multiphasic screening in the middle aged can no longer be advocated on scientific, ethical or economic grounds as a desirable public health measure'.

The two trials were relatively small, and were not without methodological problems, but the lack of a positive result was very important.

Response to the challenges

One might have expected that these significant challenges would have caused a reorientation of the theory and practice of screening, resulting in:

◆ Greater awareness amongst users of healthcare concerning the potential harm from screening, and of the incentives motivating much of its provision

◆ Far greater emphasis on evidence, with introduction of screening only once there was valid evidence that a programme resulted in more good than harm at affordable cost

◆ Re-examination and reorganization of existing screening practices where evidence was lacking

◆ Development of screening theory and of research requirements to encompass more than just test performance, and including all aspects of programme delivery and evaluation.

It actually took another 30 years of controversy and confrontation before these changes began to be taken seriously amongst the mainstream of professionals and policy makers. Things might have been different if the challenges had come sooner, but three decades of sustained promotion, in the USA and elsewhere, had had its effect. USA opinion polls by the 1960s showed broad public acceptance of periodic examination (Anderson and Rosen 1960). The public believed in the value of screening, major institutions depended on it financially and many careers had been built on the practice. The American endorsement of screening inevitably had a global effect. News travels fast, and campaign groups are quick to assume that what is best for Americans must be best for them too.

Changes did follow from the two 1968 reports and from the results of the two randomized controlled trials but, despite this, the growth of unvalidated screening showed no signs of slowing. Key changes included the following:

◆ In the UK, a formal Department of Health 'Joint Standing Subcommittee on Screening in Medical Care' was established, its first meeting taking place in January 1969. Periodic examination was not recommended. The role of the subcommittee was to give advice, but this gave no guarantee of real influence.

- Frame and Carlson in the USA published a comprehensive literature review on screening, first in 1975 (in three parts) and then updated in 1986 (Frame and Carlson 1975, parts 1, 2 and 3; Frame 1986, parts 4, 5 and 6).

- In 1976, a Canadian Task Force on the Periodic Examination was commissioned (Canadian Task Force 1979), leading to a succession of reports and recommendations concerning screening.

- In 1984. a panel was formed for the United States Preventive Services Task Force, which in 1989 published the first (US Preventive Services Task Force 1989) of a series of recommendations on screening.

What was important was that these reports took a new approach, and considered specific screening tests and their capacity to influence specific conditions, rather than considering the periodic examination as a non-specific whole. Until you define what it is you are aiming to achieve, you cannot begin to measure whether you are achieving it.

Policy making in the UK

Although the Department of Health committee, established by the Chief Medical Officer George Godber, successfully prevented the adoption in the UK of the routine general physical examination, it did not take long for the policy making processes to fall into disarray. Godber's term of office ended in 1973, and the committee survived until 1980, after which no further meetings were scheduled (Holland and Stewart 2005). Memories are short and a subsequent Minister of Health, supported then by a different Chief Medical Officer, tried to introduce routine general examinations for all adults into the family doctor contract of the late 1980s. It was only through immediate and vociferous opposition by family doctors, some of whom had been involved in the 1967 South-East London Study (see p. 16), that the policy was eventually dropped (Cook 2004). For child health screening, and cervical screening, policy and practice grew haphazardly with little link to evidence. By the 1990s, the policy making arrangements within the Department of Health were both complicated and ineffective, with gaps and overlaps that were 'wasteful and confusing; they blur responsibility and invite conflict' (Evans 1995). To solve this, a single UK Screening Committee was established in 1996, chaired by the

Chief Medical Officer Kenneth Calman. When the committee compiled an inventory of unevaluated and unregulated screening practices within the NHS, few were surprised to discover that the list ran to well over 300.

A slow but important transition had taken place between 1968 when questions were voiced only by a handful of farsighted individuals, to 1996 when the need for evidence, policy and co-ordinated delivery was gaining wider recognition. Many problems had to be overcome in order for this transition to be made. Before problems can be overcome, they first have to be recognized and acknowledged—this was not an easy matter in the politically and emotionally charged environment that screening engendered.

It is easiest to illustrate this transition with an actual case study, and for this we have used the UK cervical screening programme. We have chosen this because it was, inadvertently, a field study of what goes wrong if screening is not organized as a public health programme, and if policy is not based on evidence. The lessons are important. The story roughly follows four phases—optimism, disillusionment, organization and realism. We have simplified matters greatly and present only key events in the timeline. A basic description of the tests and interventions involved in cervical screening is given in the glossary.

Case 1.1 Case study—cervical screening in the UK, 1950—2005

In 1940s Britain, the average man or woman in the street was unlikely to have heard of cancer of the cervix. Few of us know even one person with mouth cancer, and cervix cancer in the UK had a similar frequency. Until 1950, the cervix did not even have its own code in death statistics, but was included with all cancers of the womb.

Phase one—optimism

A trans-Atlantic visit in the 1950s by an up and coming young newspaper editor helped turn cervical cancer into the familiar name that it is today. Harold Evans, prominent journalist and writer, was in his twenties when he visited the USA on a Harkness Fund Fellowship.

Case 1.1 Case study—cervical screening in the UK, 1950—2005 *(cont.)*

On returning to the UK, Evans ran a successful campaign through his paper *The Northern Echo* to get a cervical screening programme established in England. Attempts to suggest that more evidence was needed were useless. Archie Cochrane, the man whose ideas inspired Iain Chalmers to establish the now world-renowned Cochrane Collaboration, wrote in 1976 (Cochrane 1976) of the outrage that followed statements he had made in the late 1960s and early 1970s concerning the lack of evidence for cervical screening (Cochrane 1971). The response had been:

> an uproar with banner headlines attacking me in South Wales newspapers, abusive letters (some anonymous), and no colleague in Cardiff could be found to defend the 'dangerous heretic' (Cochrane 1976)

Eventually the screening service would become one of the best organized and most effective cervical cancer control campaigns anywhere in the world, but for the first 20 years of its existence it turned out to be a disaster.

Fundamental problems were:

◆ Categorization of cell and tissue changes in samples from the cervix is dependent on visual examination and is highly subjective, yet there were no uniform rules to guide classification, there was no standard training and no quality control.

◆ The cumulative age-specific incidence of new lesions in regularly screened women vastly exceeds the age-specific prevalence in newly screened women (Boyes *et al.* 1982). What this means is that the theory behind screening—that all pre-cancer progresses to cancer, and that all cancers are preceded by a detectable pre-cancerous phase—is not matched by reality. In truth, most pre-cancer is transient, and screening therefore leads to a major problem of overdiagnosis.

◆ The most appropriate screening frequency, cut-off levels for defining abnormality, interventions and means of delivering the programme to those most at risk were unknown.

Case 1.1 Case study—cervical screening in the UK, 1950—2005 *(cont.)*

- ◆ Easiest to screen were middle-class women under 35 who attended regularly for contraceptive advice or antenatal care. Yet the risk of cervix cancer is highest in older women, and those in lower socio-economic groups. The resources were therefore devoted exclusively to frequent screening of those at lowest risk.

- ◆ Hysterectomy or cone biopsy for screen-detected cervical intraepithelial neoplasia (CIN) resulted in loss of fertility in some young women still of childbearing age, and even to death from operative complications.

- ◆ Many health service staff were ambivalent about the evidence for screening, and about the wisdom of using scarce resources for cervical cytology. They were reluctant to help develop the service.

- ◆ The Department of Health failed to provide necessary central advice and leadership for such a major public health programme. Responding to campaign groups and popular opinion, they gave only the vaguest advice: 'screening should be offered to women over 35 and with special risk factors'.

Given these problems, it was not surprising that cervical screening became a battleground. The service, begun on a tide of optimism, soon became a source of major disillusionment.

Phase two—disillusionment

The numbers of tests and interventions grew massively but without any obvious impact on death rates (Knox 1982). Young low-risk women were having annual tests; older women were developing cancer and had never heard of the screening service. Some women had abnormal screening results but received no investigation, treatment or follow-up (Sharp *et al.* 1987). Only a very few localities, most notably Aberdeen in Scotland, were routinely calling up all eligible women and offering accessible services for hard to reach groups. The circumstance underpinning Aberdeen's approach was a combination of senior support from Professor Dugald Baird, plus an able and committed individual, Dr Elizabeth Macgregor, to lead on programme delivery. In most places, the service was purely a cytology testing service, not a screening programme.

Case 1.1 Case study—cervical screening in the UK, 1950—2005 *(cont.)*

Growth in facilities for colposcopy—a technique that means the cervix can be examined and treated without general anaesthetic—enabled less invasive treatments (loop excision and laser) to be used, involving only an out-patient attendance. This resulted in far more women being investigated and treated, and some even argued that all women needed colposcopy as the primary screening method.

During the 1970s and 1980s, the success or failure of all this activity was fiercely contested. Some believed that the programme must be helping simply because so many abnormalities were being found and treated. Others judged success by the mortality statistics, and concluded that the programme had failed and would continue to fail unless it was delivered very differently (Murphy *et al.* 1988). This caused an impasse. To argue for major change you have to acknowledge the problems. Yet any suggestion that the programme was not successful provoked fierce protest from those involved, partly for fear that public confidence would be lost, partly for fear that the service would be judged unimportant. George Knox, author of several key evaluations (Knox 1976, 1982; Boyes *et al.* 1982), summed up the conflict:

> It is an unfortunate fact that many questions relating to the planning and development of screening services during the last 20 years have been based on little more than a confrontation between enthusiasts and skeptics. Scientific studies—and scientific workers themselves—have often been classified as for or against, and their data and conclusions have been believed or discounted more according to the supposed category of their originators than according to their factual content and analytical validity (Knox 1982).

A turning point came in the 1980s when the death from cervix cancer of a recently screened Oxfordshire woman created a media storm. The patient had received no notification of her abnormal result, and no treatment, but this was because she had changed both her name and her address soon after she had her screening test, making it impossible for the laboratory or her family doctor to trace her. This fact was ignored in the witch hunt that followed, and most reports described the matter as an administrative error.

Case 1.1 Case study—cervical screening in the UK, 1950—2005 *(cont.)*

Importantly, this event meant that problems in the screening system could at last be acknowledged, without implying any actual limitations with screening itself. It provided an opportunity for long-standing concerns finally to gain centre stage, articulated partly through a powerful anonymous *Lancet* editorial (Anonymous 1985) written by George Knox.

The points made in Knox's 1985 editorial have general relevance for all kinds of disorganized screening, so it is worth summarizing some of them here:

◆ Since screening began in 1964, mortality from cervical cancer in England and Wales declined at 1 per cent per year, the same rate at which it seemed to be falling for several decades previously.

◆ Around 40 million tests and around 200 000 cone excisions had taken place during the 20 years, with prevention of perhaps 1000 deaths. So 40 000 tests and 200 excision biopsies happened for each life saved.

◆ The UK had only procedural objectives (to 'provide a service', not 'to reduce deaths') and no-one was in charge. Although the policy was to screen older women, it was no-one's job to see that it happened. Most tests were taken from young women, clinicians being encouraged by the fact that CIN was found in them, but the majority of CIN—Knox estimated probably over 95 per cent—are of a type that rarely progresses.

◆ National decisions about registers, computerization and responsibility for call and recall had been disastrous, making the task impossible for local programmes.

◆ Finland, Denmark, Iceland and north-east Scotland had similar expenditure but deaths had fallen. Their programmes:

were organized as public-health cancer control programmes with the explicit objective of reducing mortality, they were not simply laboratory services

called the age groups at greatest and most immediate risk (30+) and kept on trying, they concentrated first on the unscreened, and they used a population register

Case 1.1 Case study—cervical screening in the UK, 1950—2005 *(cont.)*

had someone in charge, he/she had a name and a telephone
number and could be held to account.

The editorial was a powerful stimulus to action.

Phase three—organization

Staff within the programme formed a National Co-ordinating
Network, helped by a small amount of funding from the Department
of Health. They started to streamline policies and practices across
the country, they developed training centres, defined essential
standards and performance data, and procured national computer
software. By 1988, the Department of Health was issuing proper
guidance (Department of Health and Social Security 1988), not only
about who was responsible for what, but also about how it would
be achieved. There was an official re-launch of the NHS Cervical
Screening Programme, with a national system of call and recall
operated from District registers, from April 1988. Annual statistics
were submitted by each programme, and published nationally for
all to see. By 1991, almost 90 per cent of Districts had recorded
population coverage of over 80 per cent. In 1992, the National
Audit Office produced a report on the programme (National Audit
Office 1992), and although there were still some problems, the contrast from 1985 was substantial. The success of the National Network
led to the appointment of a dedicated National Co-ordinating
Team, with responsibility for all the national cancer screening programmes (NHS Cancer Screening Programmes website).

However, the problems were not over:

◆ First, when you introduce quality improvement for a neglected
  service, you are bound to uncover serious deficiencies. This is
  indeed what happened, resulting in a succession of incidents
  and adverse publicity, starting with Inverclyde in Scotland
  where pathology standards were poor (Scottish Office 1993),
  and continuing through to the Kent and Canterbury NHS
  Trust (Wells 1997) where laboratory screeners had struggled to
  deliver a service without proper training, supervision or support
  from senior colleagues.

Case 1.1 Case study—cervical screening in the UK, 1950—2005 *(cont.)*

◆ Secondly, once screening is well delivered, this forces you to face up to its real limitations. There are some cancer cases that even good quality screening cannot prevent, and unless the limitations of screening are made explicit the staff will be blamed quite inappropriately for these cases. Also, the high rates of positive tests, most of which are transient minor cell changes, cause major anxiety unless you can change the universal belief that every abnormality must mean cancer.

Some advocated yet more fervent affirmations of the value and success of screening in order to try and conceal the limitations. This only fuels expectations to a level that can never be met. The only long-term solution is to set out what screening can achieve, and acknowledge what it cannot.

Phase four—realism

In the first half of the 1990s there were still widely differing perceptions of the cervical screening programme, depending on where people stood and what data they had access to:

◆ Outside the programme, the popular perception was that screening was a success; any problems were due to incompetence, and high rates of abnormality must be because a massive epidemic was being averted.

◆ Within the programme, the staff delivering screening had grow-ing concerns about the overdiagnosis problem and the distress this caused to hundreds of thousands of healthy women nation-wide (Anderson and Thornton 1994; Anderson 1997), but this had not been acknowledged or quantified in published literature.

◆ Death rates were not yet showing any acceleration in decline, and the shaky evidence base for the programme was eloquently summarized by critical commentators such as Petr Skrabanek (Skrabanek 1988) and James McCormick (McCormick 1989). At conferences, and in the media, this was studiously ignored, and assumptions were quoted instead, based on a guess that a life is saved for every three treatments. Such estimates were vastly different from the data quoted by Knox in 1985

Case 1.1 Case study—cervical screening in the UK, 1950—2005 *(cont.)*

(Anonymous 1985), showing 200 excisions for one benefited, and 95 per cent of CIN not progressing.

◆ Now that coverage was high, most of the cancers in women under 65 were in women who had been screened. This prompted people to insist that somehow these women had not been 'properly screened', to blame the sample takers (Macgregor *et al.* 1994) and to lower even further the thresholds for diagnosis and treatment.

Eventually the task of achieving a realistic overview, encompassing both the success and the limitations of the programme, was made possible by two publications in the *Lancet* during 1995.

◆ The first was a description of the numbers involved in an established screening programme using records since 1976 for a quarter of a million women in Bristol (Raffle *et al.* 1995). This demonstrated the extent of the overdiagnosis problem, particularly for women under 30. It showed that changing diagnostic thresholds were the major reason for the escalating detection rates.

◆ The second publication, later the same year, was an analysis of cervical cancer death rates in England and Wales (Sasieni *et al.* 1995) showing that for women born since the 1930s a new phenomenon was occurring. Previously, deaths had always risen up to age 60. In cohorts born since 1930, the deaths were now declining as the cohort aged, and in each cohort the start of the downturn took place in the late 1980s. For the first time, this gave strong evidence that the screening programme was achieving its objective.

Once there was this evidence of benefit, it became easier to gain acknowledgment that limitations existed. Official recognition of the limitations came when Sir William Wells issued the report of his inquiry panel in 1997 examining the Kent and Canterbury failings (Wells 1997). The first recommendation was:

> There should be better information nationally about the advantages and limitations of the screening test as well as a national publicity strategy to improve understanding of the screening programme (Kent and Canterbury Inquiry, Wells 1997).

Case 1.1 Case study—cervical screening in the UK, 1950—2005 *(cont.)*

Within a few years this was reflected in the national policies for the programme (NHS Cervical Screening Programme 2001).

In due course sense began to be made of the confusing and apparently opposing opinions surrounding screening (Slater 1998). The notion that screening was neither wonderful nor useless, but somewhere in between, gained ground. The nationally led approach of rigorous quality assurance reached all parts of the system and all localities, with the result that the entire population was served by a comprehensive and accessible programme delivered by well trained staff and encompassing efficient call, recall, follow-up and failsafe systems. Subsequent analyses (Quinn *et al.* 1999, Sasieni and Adams 1999) gave more detailed estimates of lives saved, and the Bristol data could be set alongside these mortality models in order to derive an overall analysis of benefits, harms and progression rates (Raffle *et al.* 2003).

Since then, the discourse around screening has steadily become more balanced and more calm as each year goes by, resulting in far more productive debate than was possible a few decades ago.

This example describes a slow transition from a haphazard and largely ineffective activity begun on a wave of unrealistic optimism, to a well-ordered programme that met realistic objectives. Numerous countries have tackled these problems, for a diverse range of screening activities. Holland and Stewart, in their recent book summarize current approaches to screening in six European countries, revealing astonishing differences between nations in public acceptance of the range and quality of screening provision (Holland and Stewart 2005). The case study above illustrates, for one programme and for one nation, the types of problem that have to be solved if you want screening to deliver a cost-effective public health programme. The ideal is to avoid these problems in the first place, by gathering evidence before deciding to introduce a programme, and by planning screening as a system, with integral quality controls. This is easier said than done, and even when it is achieved plenty of dilemmas remain.

Post-modern screening

> Postmodernism is a contemporary movement. It is strong and fashionable.
> Over and above this, it is not altogether clear what the devil it is. In fact,
> clarity is not conspicuous amongst its marked attributes …; the notion that
> everything is a 'text', that the basic material of texts, societies and almost
> anything is meaning, that meanings are there to be decoded or 'decon-
> structed', that the notion of objective reality is suspect—all this seems to be
> part of the atmosphere, or mist, in which postmodernism flourishes, or
> which postmodernism helps to spread.
>
> Ernest Gellner (1992)

So here we are in the twenty-first century. The modern approach to
screening, articulated in the 1960s by Holland, Cochrane, Wilson and
Jungner, Knox, McKeown and many more, eventually made an impact.

- Before the 1950s we had 'pre-modern' screening, founded on a
  supreme confidence in the beneficial power of science, technology
  and medicine.

- In the 1960s, this confidence was challenged and the 'modern'
  screening era began, based on rationalism, evidence, organization,
  economic evaluation, and an ethical duty to be certain that good
  exceeded harm.

The limits of rationalism

However, the world has moved on. Modern screening was decided by
experts, delivered as a utilitarian programme and complied with by
dutiful and grateful patients. Post-modern screening will operate in
societies very different from those of the 1960s, and screening will
have to adapt. Some of the likely influences are:

- New pressures arising from the need to conserve natural resources
  and mitigate and adapt to climate change—the effects this will
  have on political, economic and health systems are unpredictable,
  but are likely to be far reaching (Martin 2006)

- Declining medical, scientific and expert authority

- Heightened expectations for the elimination of risk

- Rights of patients to receive full and balanced information, to
  appeal against policy and decisions, and to seek legal redress

- Growing availability of tests relating to genetic factors

- Transition away from centralized state-organized provision of services
- Tensions around funding and affordability of healthcare.

We will return to some of these themes in Chapter 8 when we look at how screening policy is made. However, first we need to work through the theory and practice of defining, evaluating and delivering screening, which we cover in Chapters 2–7.

Summary points

The idea of routinely examining healthy people was proposed as long ago as 1861 by Horace Dobell in London. George Gould in the USA developed the idea, primarily with the aim of improving scientific knowledge about disease and its prevention.

In the USA, the practice of routine health examination grew because of a combination of factors, unrelated to any definitive evidence that this led to more good than harm or was a valuable use of resources.

The driving factors in the USA were the insurance companies' need to minimize financial risk, the employers need to guard against claims and ensure a healthy workforce, the medical profession's need to avoid having their role usurped by state healthcare, and healthcare plan providers' need to control unfettered demand for health checks.

In the UK, the only routine screening before the 1950s was medical and dental checks for children, instigated in 1904 partly in response to fears of growing military strength in Germany.

Concerns from rigorously minded academics led to challenges in the 1960s, in the form of two authoritative reports and the instigation of two randomized controlled trials of multiphasic health examinations, neither of which showed benefit to general health or mortality.

From 1960, there was growing acceptance of the need to evaluate benefit and harms from screening, together with recognition of the importance of quality-assured programme delivery and the ethical duty to provide balanced information.

> **Summary points** *(cont.)*
>
> The rational approach to screening is likely to face challenges in the future, due to a diminution of traditional authority vested in medicine and science, changing perception of the need to control risk, increasing use of genetic tests, reduction in centralized provision of healthcare and tensions about healthcare funding.

Test yourself

Question one

In the 1960s concerns began to be raised about screening by those who argued for a more rational approach, most notably through the World Health Organization booklet (Wilson and Jungner 1968) and the Nuffield Trust essays (Nuffield Provincial Hospitals Trust 1968) (see p 10). Which of the following were factors contributing to those concerns? (mark each of the following as yes or no)

(a) Not enough screening was directed at infants.

(b) Screening was being introduced into routine practice before being properly evaluated.

(c) Screening was only offered for rare diseases.

(d) Screening was being offered to healthy subjects without explaining the uncertainties and the potential for harm; this was unethical.

(e) There was a widespread assumption that screening must be automatically beneficial irrespective of any clear evidence of improved outcomes.

(f) The insistence on evidence was causing unacceptable delays to the adoption of new screening procedures.

(g) Screening was saving a great deal of money and needed to be more widely implemented.

(h) Authoritative bodies were making sweeping recommendations about screening, based not on evidence but on professional opinion.

(i) Members of the public were being persuaded to campaign for screening interventions that could lead to more harm than good.

(j) Public funds were being diverted away from activities of certain benefit in order to fund screening procedures which were not proved and were possibly harmful.

Question two

In the case study of cervical screening in the UK (see p. 19), can you list some of the differences between the screening that was provided in the 1970s and that led to so much disillusionment, compared with the screening provided by the late 1990s once all the lessons were learnt?

Chapter 2

What screening is, and is not

The aim of the chapter

The aim of this chapter is to review the different ways in which the term 'screening' has been and is used, and to define the meaning that we will use throughout the rest of the book.

In the first chapter we described some of the scientific, political and commercial factors that shaped the growth of screening over the past century. This growth led to the range of established activities that we now think of as health screening or medical screening. These activities vary widely in purpose and process, encompassing bloodspot tests in newborn babies, questions asked of older people to screen for dementia, or whole-body scans, using computerized tomography (CT) or magnetic resonance imaging (MRI), for the wealthy worried well. In this chapter we define screening by using, and building on, the existing definitions. We explain the different kinds of testing done on healthy people, and how these differ from diagnostic tests done to solve the problems patients bring to clinicians. We explain where screening fits in the pathway of disease development and we describe the basic system needed if screening is successfully to achieve risk reduction.

Definitions and meanings

Most of us give little thought to the difference between a definition and a meaning, yet philosophers have devoted years of deliberation to these questions. Ludwig Wittgenstein, one of the most influential philosophers of the twentieth century, held that words do not have 'right' meanings they simply have uses. Some uses are clearer than others and some are newer than others. Our failure to clarify and agree what we mean by the terms we use is the cause of many, indeed Wittgenstein believed all, disagreements (Kenny 2005).

Clarity about use of terms is important, since the way people use the term screening varies widely across the globe, across different professional groups and across time. Definitions do not necessarily capture these subtleties and variations.

What we mean by screening

The universal features of activities described as screening are:

- People being screened either do not have or have not recognized the signs or symptoms of the condition being tested for. In other words, they believe themselves to be well in relation to the disease that the screening relates to

- The purpose, explicitly or implicitly, is either:

  - to reduce risk of future ill health, e.g. when adults are screened for raised blood pressure, intervention involves treatment with drugs and risk of stroke is reduced, or

  - to give information, even though risk cannot be changed, e.g. when a pregnant woman who would not contemplate termination of pregnancy chooses to be screened for Down's syndrome; if the baby is found to have Down's syndrome the parents are forewarned.

These features relate to the context, and not to any specific attributes of the test.

The screen is a sieving process to find a few from amongst many.

Box 2.1 Dictionary definition

The *Shorter Oxford English Dictionary* defines the verb 'to screen' as: 'to sift by passing through a screen'. This definition, first noted in 1664, is only one of six, the others referring to screens without holes such as, for example, a cinema screen. The verb 'to sift' derives, like the word 'sieve', from an old Dutch word *zeef*, for 'a utensil consisting of a circular frame with a finely meshed or perforated bottom, used to separate the coarser from the finer particles of any loose material'.

The initial test does not in itself give a definitive answer. Instead it separates two main groups, those told their test is negative and those told their test is positive. The group with a positive result then needs further scrutiny to sort out who is likely to benefit from being offered intervention.

Formal definitions of screening

A main source of confusion in the everyday use of the term 'screening' is that it can mean any of the following:

◆ A screening test offered opportunistically to one person

◆ A screening test offered systematically to a group of people or a whole population

◆ A set of loosely linked activities encompassing screening tests and interventions that roughly comprise a screening programme

◆ A rigorously quality-assured and evidence-based screening programme encompassing all necessary steps for achievement of risk reduction.

We believe that all of these activities may be screening of one sort or another.

There are various formal definitions for screening, and these too vary over the matter of whether screening refers to tests or programmes, and to individuals or populations. In this book, we focus on screening programmes, aimed at risk reduction for the screened individual, based on sound evidence and delivered to pre-agreed policy and standards. Across the world, the way in which such programmes are achieved varies widely, from centralized arrangements where staff are directly employed by a single organization, through to provision by multiple independent practitioners and agencies but following common procedures.

Table 2.1 shows three formal definitions of screening. The US Commission definition is more concerned with tests than with the whole programme, whereas the two UK definitions define screening as a systematic, or public health activity, and focus on what screening should be, rather than what screening sometimes is. All definitions include the hallmark that subjects do not have, or have not

Table 2.1 Formal definitions of screening

US Commission on Chronic Illness 1957 (Commission Chronic Illness 1957)	The presumptive identification of unrecognized disease or defect by the application of tests, examinations or other procedures which can be applied rapidly. Screening tests sort out apparently well persons who probably have a disease from those who probably do not. A screening test is not intended to be diagnostic. Persons with positive or suspicious findings must be referred to their physicians for diagnosis and necessary treatment.
Journal of Medical Screening 1994 (Wald 1994)	Screening is the systematic application of a test or inquiry, to identify individuals at sufficient risk of a specific disorder to benefit from further investigation or direct preventive action, among persons who have not sought medical attention on account of symptoms of that disorder.
UK National Screening Committee (2000)	Screening is a public health service in which members of a defined population who do not necessarily perceive they are at risk of or already affected by a disease or complications are asked a question or offered a test, to identify those individuals who are more likely to be helped than harmed by further tests or treatments to reduce the risk of a disease or its complications.

recognized, any signs or symptoms, and the fact that screening deals with probabilities not certainties. The UK definitions mention that screening should confer greater chance of benefit than harm.

It is interesting to look back at the 1968 Nuffield Essays (see also Chapter 1, p. 10) to see how the term 'screening' was defined and used then. McKeown's introductory chapter in the essays (McKeown 1968) stated that they interpreted screening as: 'a medical investigation which does not arise from a patient's request for advice for specific complaints'.

This definition would cause confusion today as many screening examinations arise directly as a result of individual requests because of the immense publicity about possible screening tests and disease risks. In this instance, the person requesting screening does not have a specific sign or symptom, but some would argue that their heightened worry about risk could constitute a 'complaint'. This is a practical illustration of how meanings, usages and definitions change with time.

McKeown also subdivided screening according to its aims, with the three groups being research, public protection and direct contribution to the health of the screened individual, which he termed 'prescriptive screening'. This third group is the use we are primarily concerned with in this book.

At this point, we should also note that sometimes a test or investigation done for one purpose, for example to check if there is a pelvic bone fracture after a fall, can turn out to be a screening test for another condition, by showing, for example, that the patient has an aortic aneurysm. The patient did not consent to this screening test but, once the information is uncovered, there is no going back. This can pose significant dilemmas when the value of intervention is uncertain. A healthy person may, for example, end up having their oesophagus surgically removed to prevent a possible future cancer, because an endoscopy for a different reason lead to a biopsy showing the presence of possible cancer cells. In cases such as this, the evidence that benefit outweighs harm is non-existent, the patient gave no consent for being screened for cancer, but in effect the test became a screening procedure almost by accident.

Box 2.2 Our definition of what screening is

To summarize all this, we take screening to mean:

- ◆ Testing of people who either do not have or have not recognized the signs or symptoms of the condition being tested for. In other words, they believe themselves to be well in relation to the disease that the screening relates to.

- ◆ Where the stated or implied purpose is to reduce risk for that individual of future ill health in relation to the condition being tested for, or to give information about risk that is deemed valuable for that individual even though risk cannot be altered.

- ◆ It encompasses the whole system or programme of events necessary to achieve risk reduction. Screening is a programme not a test.

Where screening fits in the disease pathway

Screening aims to identify people at an earlier stage in a disease's natural history than if they presented with symptoms. There are many steps on the pathway from health to serious disease. Factors to do with the host (the individual person) and their environment (e.g. exposure to cancer-causing agents) play a role at each stage. These factors influence whether, and how fast, the biological changes progress to more serious disease, or whether they revert to normal or are kept in check by the body's own defence mechanisms and therefore do not progress to manifest disease. Figure 2.1 illustrates a simplified version of the type of process we are talking about.

To help to understand and visualize this process, think of the fact that a risk marker for heart disease (high serum cholesterol) and pathological changes in blood vessel walls (fatty streaks) have been detected in infants. These infants will not actually develop symptomatic heart disease until many decades later, and some may not develop manifest disease in their lifetime.

It is not unusual to hear people talk about screening as though it can be applied at all these stages. This is misleading, because screening describes the sieving process applied to people before they get symptoms. Table 2.2 summarizes the contribution of screening.

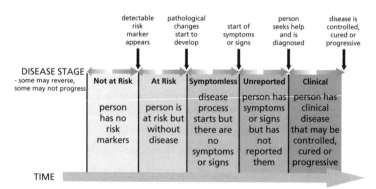

Fig. 2.1 Stages in the disease pathway.

Table 2.2 Where screening fits in the disease pathway

Stage in the natural history of disease	Contribution of screening
Person at risk: no pathological changes present	Screening for risk marker
Pathologically definable change present: symptomless stage	Screening for pathological change
Signs and/or symptoms present but disease undiagnosed	Campaigns to raise awareness of disease and encourage earlier presentation of symptoms or signs—these are sometimes called screening but are actually prompt recognition. Surveillance to look for unrecognized signs or symptoms, e.g. at child health clinics.
Clinical phase	Individuals with a particular disease may receive routine tests as part of clinical management. This is sometimes called screening but is usually concerned with controlling the disease, the side effects of treatment or with diagnosing and managing associated conditions.

Other kinds of testing in people without signs or symptoms

We have explained that in this book we are focusing on screening programmes that bring benefit to the screened individual either through achieving reduction in risk from the disease being screened for, or occasionally through giving information that is important for the individual even though risk cannot be changed.

There are more reasons for testing healthy people than the reasons covered by our definition. Here are some examples. They have many of the characteristics of screening, but they also have important differences from the type of health screening that we are considering in this book.

◆ *Insurance medicals.* These give information for insurance companies to enable them to set appropriate premiums for life-insurance policies.

- *Employment checks.* These protect people who could be affected by the employee, for example lorry drivers need eyesight checks in order to gain their driving licence, teachers and healthcare workers are checked for tuberculosis (TB) to ensure that schoolchildren and patients are not at risk of catching TB.

- *Safety checks.* Patients undergoing general anaesthesia may have an electrocardiogram ordered by the anaesthetist, and patients commencing a drug known to be toxic to the liver will have liver function tests done before they start the treatment. These tests are not being performed for diagnosis, but nor are they screening. They give information that increases the chance of a safe anaesthetic, or the chance of spotting quickly if liver damage is occurring so that the drug treatment can then be altered.

- *Infection control.* People in contact with known cases of communicable diseases such as TB or syphilis are recommended to have tests, partly for their own benefit but partly to avoid further onward transmission. There are important differences between infection control testing and classic screening programmes. Testing is only one component of any infectious disease control programme, and strategies for control will depend on characteristics such as mode of transmission, infectivity, incubation period, severity, existence of carriers and vectors, on the availability of immunization or other measures, and on social and cultural factors. Public health legislation exists that gives powers to restrict the freedoms of individuals who are putting others at risk. Infection control programmes are beyond the scope of this book.

- *Epidemiological research.* Population studies often involve testing in healthy subjects, for example to determine disease prevalence, or to examine risk factors and their relationship to subsequent outcome. Participants give informed consent, and protocols determine action that should or should not take place in the event of potentially serious risk factors or disease being discovered. The aim is to gather data that will improve knowledge and understanding of health and disease.

- *Lifestyle checks and fitness testing.* These tests are done usually as a first step in trying to improve general health and fitness. They can act as a motivator, a benchmark for measuring improvement, and can help determine what advice and what sort of physical activity is appropriate for that person. They are health promotion, not screening.

- ◆ *Testing for associated conditions.* Sometimes the presence of one disorder makes it likely that another condition may also occur, for example the skin disorder acanthosis nigris is associated with bowel cancer. Diagnostic testing is needed to confirm or rule out the presence of the associated condition because a screening test will not give a certain enough answer. So in this example, a patient with acanthosis nigris should be offered colonoscopy, not just faecal occult blood testing.

Screening is ethically different from clinical practice

Population thinking versus individual thinking

Sometimes screening provokes fierce controversy. Public health practitioners are reluctant to implement screening until they have robust evidence, and until a comprehensive quality-assured programme can be put in place. They frequently find themselves in conflict with clinicians or members of the public who are angry that screening is not already provided. Why is it that clinicians and public health practitioners can have such different viewpoints on screening?

Clinicians are faced daily with patients who they believe could have been helped by screening. Members of the public may have had relatives affected by illness they think could have been prevented, or may themselves have had a screening test and feel they owe their lives to it. Clinicians and individual patients are familiar with the notion that a treatment brings a risk of side effects. They are used to accepting the possibility that an individual will fall into one of the groups in Table 2.3.

Every patient hopes they will be in group A, accepts that they might finish up in either group B or group C, and tries to ignore the possibility that they could finish up in group D, having side effects without any beneficial effect. They will want access to the treatment because for them it brings a chance of benefit. If others who take it are harmed, that does not matter to them.

Table 2.3 Individual risk of benefit and harm from treatment

		Beneficial effects of treatment	
		Benefit	*No benefit*
Harmful effects of treatment	*No harm*	A. Treatment helps, no side effects	B. Treatment does not help, no side effects
	Harm	C. Treatment helps, and brings side effects	D. Treatment does not help, but brings side effects

The same applies when an individual considers having a screening test, for example for detecting localized prostate cancer. The prostate test is a blood test known as the prostate-specific antigen (PSA) test. As long as the individual believes there is a chance, no matter how small, of deriving benefit, then they may well want the test.

Current available evidence shows that PSA testing will harm far more men, through the side effects of invasive investigations and treatments, than it could help (this is explained in more detail in Chapters 4, 7, and 8). So a public health practitioner, whose 'patient' is the whole population, will be interested in the overall harm and the overall benefit, not just in whether there is a theoretical chance of someone being helped. He or she will want to protect the population from PSA screening because of the overall harm.

Therefore, these different perspectives explain why some clinicians and members of the public feel that screening should be provided even when there is no evidence of benefit, whereas the public health practitioner who has looked at the evidence wants to avoid the harms of screening being visited on his or her population. The public health practitioner's view will be vigorously opposed by those campaigning for screening on the grounds that it is an individual's right.

Principles of screening

Screening should involve a system not just a test

All three of the definitions shown in Table 2.1 refer to the fact that further action is necessary once risk is identified. The second and third definitions mention that screening should be systematic. We should always aim to deliver screening as a well-organized system if we want to achieve more benefit than harm.

This does not mean that *ad hoc* and haphazard testing for symptomless people falls completely outside the definition of screening. For example, consider the case of Mrs Smith, a 50-year-old woman with no signs or symptoms of heart disease who receives an exercise electrocardiogram as part of a whole-body screen at a private clinic. If an abnormality is found, she will be given the result and it will be up to her to seek further investigation and possible treatment. Evidence about the consequences of exercise electrocardiography in people without signs or symptoms of heart disease shows that it is a very poor screening test, leading to more harm than good (Gibbons *et al.* 2002) (questions two and three at the end of Chapter 4 give a bit more detail about this). So the screening that Mrs Smith is receiving involves only a test and not a programme, and it is not based on evidence. Yet it is still screening, because she is healthy and the implied promise is future risk reduction from heart disease.

In this book, we want to look at screening as the whole system by which you achieve improved health. Identification of risk cannot change outcome unless an intervention follows and, conversely, specific interventions for higher risk individuals cannot happen without widespread application of some initial test or inquiry to capture those at higher risk.

Box 2.3 You can't have one without the other

Identification of risk or symptomless disease and effective intervention to reduce risk or treat symptomless disease are inextricably linked. You cannot intervene unless you identify, and there is little point identifying unless you intervene effectively.

Many years of frustrating experience showed that if you regard screening as simply doing the tests, then you are unlikely to achieve much real improvement in the public's health. One example is the case study about cervical cytology testing (see Chapter 1, p. 19). Another is the very early experience with testing by health visitors to screen for phenylketonuria (PKU) in newborn babies.

Case 2.1 Case study—phenylketonuria screening: development of a system

Phenylketonuria (PKU) is a rare inherited disorder that some babies are born with. A specific liver enzyme, phenylalinine hydroxylase, is lacking, which means that one particular protein component in food, phenylalanine, cannot be processed and it builds up in the tissues. Most, but not all, of the affected children develop brain damage resulting in severe learning difficulties. Early recognition of the condition, and adherence to a special diet low in phenylalanine, can enable normal brain development and intelligence. As with many conditions, the disease is 'heterogeneous', which means that the degree of enzyme deficiency varies from case to case.

Introduction of PKU screening for all newborn babies was not entirely straightforward (Wilson 1968), largely because of lack of certain evidence concerning natural history across the spectrum of disease and concerning the impact of intervention. There were legitimate concerns that all PKU-detected children would be subjected to a very unpalatable and restrictive diet throughout their childhood, with a potential adverse impact on behavioural and social development, yet it was possible that some of these children with a milder degree of PKU would have had normal intelligence even with a normal diet. Other concerns included uncertainty about how strictly and for how long the diet was needed, and concerns about brain damage in babies in the next generation unless mothers with PKU resumed the diet before and during their pregnancies. Enactment of legislation in many States of the USA made PKU screening compulsory, although some felt this was premature and that more research into dietary management was needed (Bessman 1966).

In 1963, the UK Ministry of Health commended, through the Chief Medical Officer's letter to Medical Officers of Health (Ministry of Health 1963), the recommendations from the Medical Research Council conference of 1960 advising urine testing by health visitors when infants were 4–6 weeks old. This test used a Phenistix pressed onto a wet nappy and if the colour changed to bluish green this

Case 2.1 Case study—phenylketonuria screening: development of a system *(cont.)*

was positive. In 1959, in Birmingham, UK, the health visiting service conducted a survey to test all babies, and this revealed four positive tests in 19 000 babies (Ferrer 1968). This seemed reasonable based on what was known about the likely incidence of PKU at that time, and the Birmingham health visiting service continued to test the urine of all babies routinely in order to pick up cases of PKU. Recent data have shown that the incidence of PKU is around one in 12 000 births (Sanderson *et al.* 2006). For an individual health visitor, PKU is so rare that it would be at most a once in a lifetime occurrence to find a positive case. A sample of urine from an untreated case was therefore kept in the refrigerator so that the health visitors could refresh their memories of what a positive result looked like (Ferrer 1968).

During the subsequent years, however, the pick up rate in Birmingham was very low, with only three positive cases detected in the 126 000 babies tested during 1960–1965. Clinical diagnosis of PKU continued to occur, despite the fact that in theory these cases should have been picked up by the health visitor testing. Two factors probably contributed to this: first is that we now know that the urine test has poor sensitivity in newborns due to the immaturity of the liver enzymes, second is the difficulty for the health visitors when they have no regular experience of positive cases. It may be that when cases did occur, the health visitor possibly did not notice the colour change, or possibly did not believe it, or possibly the significance was not appreciated and the observation was just noted but no action taken.

During the late 1960s and early 1970s, many countries introduced centralized laboratory testing using heel prick bloodspot tests, and this took place in the UK around 1969. The laboratories performed many tens of thousands of tests, which meant that regular positives became an expected occurrence for staff. Laboratories were also well used to operating quality checks on all their work, and the pick up of PKU now became successful. Senior staff in the screening laboratories made sure that the babies with a positive test were referred in a timely manner for appropriate diagnostic investigations and clinical follow-up. After that, clinical services were developed

> **Case 2.1 Case study—phenylketonuria screening: development of a system** *(cont.)*
>
> for children with PKU, and their families, so they could receive appropriate advice and ongoing support for the management of their condition. The girls were given advice and support relating to resumption of a restricted diet if they were planning a pregnancy. Even now there are still some deficiencies in the provision of services for PKU in some parts of the UK, with some parts of the system having insufficient resources. What this case study illustrates is that provision of a testing service, as happened in the early 1960s in Birmingham, is unlikely to achieve much. For screening to deliver a real improvement in health, it needs to be a fully fledged system with all the components in place, working to high standards, and linked together.

Therefore, if you are serious about achieving best outcomes for a population, it is essential to think in terms of screening systems, not screening tests, with a system being defined as a set of activities with a common set of objectives. The system, or programme as it is more commonly known, consists of all activities, from identifying and informing those to be offered screening through to the treatment and follow-up of those found to have abnormality, and support for those who develop disease despite screening.

What does a screening system consist of?

There are two ways of looking at a screening system. One is to look at all the things that someone running a screening programme needs to have in place in order for the screened individuals to receive a good quality, reliable, supportive, effective service. This is like a map of the programme.

At this stage, all we want to do is to show you the diagram in Fig. 2.2 to introduce the concept of what has to be in place to deliver high quality screening. We have called this a 'programme map' because it shows everything that you need to worry about when you are making sure

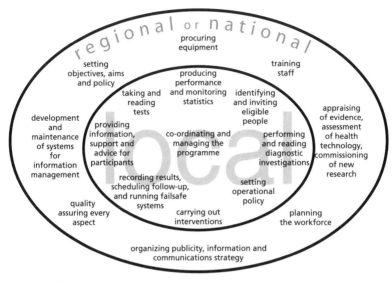

Fig. 2.2 Programme map.

that high quality screening is available to your local resident population. Later, in Chapters 5, 6 and 7, we return to this in more detail when we work through the practical issues of delivering quality-assured screening. The items in the central oval are the core activities in the programme, which are likely to be the responsibility of local organizations. The items in the outer area are essential supporting activities, and it may be that national or regional bodies will look after these aspects. We have not attempted to join any of these activities with lines, because of the huge variation that exists between different programmes, and different healthcare systems, regarding the organizational arrangements for service delivery, accountability and quality control. Suffice it to say that where there is delivery of a high quality screening programme, someone somewhere is doing each of these activities to a greater or lesser extent, and constructive relationships and communication exist between the different elements of the system.

The other way of looking at screening is to consider the steps that the screened individual goes through. This looks like a flow diagram.

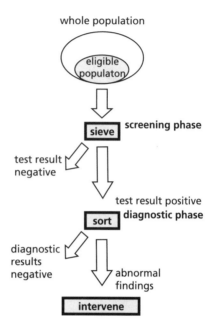

Fig. 2.3 Basic screening flow diagram.

The basic steps in a screening programme for reducing disease risk in a population are as shown in Fig. 2.3.

It is helpful to think of the initial screening process as a 'sieve', and any subsequent testing and investigation as a 'sort'. Later we use the term 'reassure' to mean telling people that their screening test or subsequent diagnostic test has a negative result. People will be reassured by this information, but they should be clear that this is not a guarantee that they do not have, or will not develop, the disease at some time in the future.

Anyone with experience of delivering screening will realize that this diagram is an oversimplification, because it misses out equivocal results, and categories that fall in between 'reassurance' and 'intervention'. It is an idealized version of screening. The inevitable uncovering of uncertain categories of disease is a constant problem in screening, and one that has been given insufficient recognition and attention in the past. Often, when a proposed new programme is at the planning stage, the issue of equivocal results and uncertain categories gets dismissed as though it will not apply. Establishing a clear and agreed case definition for the condition being screened for is an essential and difficult part of planning, evaluating and delivering screening. Even with a clear case definition, it is usual to find that the apparent incidence in the population of the condition being screened for rises once screening is in practice. This is because cases that would not have been clinically apparent are being added to the diagnosed group. This is a crucially important issue, and we explain it in more detail in Chapters 3 and 4.

Those with experience in screening will also recognize that because there are many different screening programmes, some do not precisely fit the pathway shown in Fig. 2.3. With some screening, chlamydia testing for example, there is no separate sorting phase, and intervention is offered according to the result of the initial test. With antenatal screening you are concerned with the health of parent and infant, and the issues may be too complex to summarize with this one diagram.

System outcomes matter, not just test performance

In the early days of screening, people tended to focus solely on measures of how well the screening test performed. The classic measures of test performance are sensitivity, specificity, positive predictive value and receiver operator characteristic curves. These measures are explained fully in Chapter 4, but a simple explanation of sensitivity and specificity is given here for ease of reference. Sensitivity and specificity are measures of the ability of a test to identify correctly cases as cases, and non-cases as non-cases. Case definition is of critical importance. A test of blood cholesterol detects raised blood cholesterol, and the case definition is confirmed raised blood cholesterol defined for example by a repeat test, or by a split sample tested in a reference laboratory. The test sensitivity tells you nothing about the ability of the test to predict accurately those destined to suffer a heart attack that could be prevented by lifestyle changes or medication.

Box 2.4 Sensitivity and specificity

Sensitivity is the ability of a test to identify correctly cases as positive.

Specificity is the ability of a test to identify correctly non-cases as negative.

So, the measures of test performance tell us how well the sieving phase matches the sorting phase but they ignore the steps that follow after, and it is these steps that actually determine how much benefit and harm screening brings. We have to think in terms of system performance, not just test performance. By and large this is now widely accepted, but regrettably there are still attempts to justify screening, with PSA testing or with new genetic tests, for example, purely on the basis of test performance.

It is obviously important to know whether you have a screening test that accurately predicts the results of diagnostic testing, or in other words has high sensitivity and specificity, but on its own this is not enough. You also have to be certain that:

* The cases you pick up on screening definitely would have developed serious disease or died of the condition, and that earlier detection improves the outcome. In Chapter 4 we consider the evidence we need in order to be sure of this.

* The programme can be properly organized to achieve consistent quality standards so that the desired outcomes, demonstrated in research trials, can be achieved by ordinary services. In Chapters 5 and 6 we consider how this is done.

Different models of delivery and funding

The way that screening is funded and delivered varies considerably from one programme to another and from one healthcare system to another. There may be:

* State funding and provision of approved quality-assured national programmes. This is the situation in many countries for newborn screening. In the UK, it applies currently for all programmes, although aspects of the service, for example the printing and despatch of letters, may be delivered under contract from independent companies. Family doctors in the UK are independent self-employed practitioners and provide many of the testing services. Virtually all their remuneration is from the NHS, and controls of quality and practice are uniformly applied.

* State reimbursement for recommended screening activities, with independent or state providers delivering and regulating the service.

This is the situation in Australia for example for a number of adult screening programmes.

♦ Authoritative recommendations to consumers as to what screening is advised, and the consumer decides whether they can afford an insurance policy that includes the screening activity. This is the situation for adult screening programmes in the USA.

Our own involvement in screening has primarily been in the UK NHS. It is worth explaining some of the specific features of the NHS that lend themselves to the delivery of national programmes, although these features are by no means unique to the UK.

♦ Every resident is entitled to register with a family doctor close to where they live and all but a tiny minority do so. The family doctor practice delivers services to each registered patient according to national policy and standards, organizes access to specialist services and ensures continuity of care.

♦ The family doctor registration records are held on a nationwide database, administered at county level but with uniform national software and linkages. This provides a central call and recall list used for screening programmes.

♦ Every registered birth is entered onto a dedicated child health computer system covering the administrative area, again with uniform national software and linkages between areas. This is used for newborn and infant screening so covers all children whether registered with a family doctor or not.

♦ Performance statistics for screening are compiled using uniform reports from every locality and collated into annual nationally published statistical bulletins (Department of Health Publications and Statistics website 2006).

♦ National policy for screening is formulated through the National Screening Programmes and the National Screening Committee. Information about national policy and the evidence upon which this is based is available through the National Library for Health (NHS National Library for Health, Screening Specialist Sublibrary 2006) and through the NHS Screening Programmes website. A comprehensive and valuable resume of policy and current issues is given in Holland and Stewart (2005).

Within every healthcare system, some screening takes place despite the fact that it is not endorsed or recommended by any authoritative body. One example is whole-body scans for screening healthy subjects using CT or MRI. This type of activity happens either in a private arrangement, which the client pays for directly, or as a service arranged by employers, or occasionally by public agencies when enthusiastic clinicians feel that a test is worthwhile.

Screening that fits the definition of testing healthy people with the aim of risk reduction is spread across a whole continuum according to:

♦ how closely or not it conforms with the goal of being based on sound evidence, and

♦ the extent to which it is delivered as a co-ordinated and quality assured total programme.

Genetics and screening

Since Watson and Crick's famous discovery in 1953 of the double helix structure of DNA, and more recently the sequencing of the entire human genome, there have been immense advances in understanding the structure of genes. This has fuelled great hopes for genetic engineering of new drugs, for genetic screening and for gene therapy.

In the past, 'genetics' was concerned predominantly with single-gene disorders. These are generally rare diseases caused by a variation (a mutation) in a single gene. Inheritance follows the traditional 'Mendelian' pattern. Examples of single-gene disorders include Huntington's disease and Duchenne muscular dystrophy. Where tests are used for these disorders these are generally for diagnosis, though as we shall see these can be administered in symptomless individuals who, by virtue of their family history, are at high risk of developing the disorder. Such tests, and the care and support for dealing with the consequences, are often administered by specialized medical geneticists.

As genetic research and molecular biology has progressed, more has been learned about the almost ubiquitous role of genetic factors in common disorders. This has led to the introduction of the term 'complex genetic disorders'. Here illness, rather than being caused by clear-cut defects in genes, depends upon the combined effect of several or even many 'risk variants' of genes, each of which alone confers only a small increase in risk of illness. Any one of the risk variants associated with the condition could be relatively common in the population, but most people who have them will not actually develop disease as a result. It is only the co-existence of a certain combination of risk variants and other non-genetic factors that results in disease. Our knowledge about the entire pattern needed is often incomplete. For example, risk variants involved in lipid metabolism and tissue repair are known to be involved in Alzheimer's disease, but are common in the population. Genetic screening for these variants would be useless for predicting the likelihood of Alzheimer's in an individual (Liddell *et al.* 2001). This is because it would give no greater accuracy than predictions based on age and family history alone.

The special feature of tests that relate to variations in genes, whether they are being used for diagnosis or for screening, is that the result of the test can have implications for individuals other than the person accepting a test. For example, you might test Mr Brown in Sheffield, and find a result that shows that Mr Brown's brother who lives in Australia is likely to be a genetic carrier for a disorder that could result in any children he has being seriously affected. This raises issues about what to do with this knowledge, when the brother in Australia did not know of or consent to the testing. Another way in which the results of genetic tests affect others is by revealing non-paternity. In other words, a test can reveal that the person who believed he was the father of a child is not in fact the father.

Because of the nature of genetic disorders, genetic testing is particularly important in families with known single-gene disorders. Where couples have a very high risk of conceiving an affected baby it is possible to offer *in vitro* fertilization (IVF) with testing of the resulting embryos before implantation. Only unaffected embryos are then implanted. This is known as 'pre-implantation genetic testing'. Alternatively, genetic testing can be performed when a foetus is in the uterus, to see if a specific disorder has been inherited. Also newborn babies may be tested to see if they need therapy, and adults may be tested to predict whether they are likely to develop symptomatic disease later in life. The individuals being tested are at known high risk, and this is not screening. In effect, the screening step was the inquiry that established the existence of affected individuals in the family, and the tests are to establish a diagnosis in an embryo, child or adult.

The language and terminology surrounding genetics and genetic testing is complex and potentially confusing for the non-specialist. There are numerous genetic tests and many ways in which they are used. A definition of genetic testing is 'the analysis of human DNA, RNA, chromosomes, proteins and certain metabolites in order to detect heritable disease-related genotypes, mutations, phenotypes or karyotypes for clinical purposes' (Holtzman and Watson 1999). This definition itself requires most of us to reach for the dictionary before we can fully understand it.

It is important not to be put off by the technical jargon surrounding the subject of genetics. Where screening is concerned you still need to ask the basic questions:

- What is your aim, what adverse outcome are you going to reduce the risk of?
- What is it you are actually testing for, what does the test actually measure, what is your case definition?
- Do you know what the natural course of disease would be in all cases?
- What are all the potential consequences for the tested individual, what are the consequences for other family members who have not been tested?
- Where is the evidence that benefit exceeds harm, and is the cost affordable?
- Who are you going to offer testing to, what does the whole screening programme consist of?
- How will you ensure informed choice?
- How will you guarantee the quality of the programme?

A starting point for finding out about specific tests is the National Institutes for Health database of genetic tests at the GeneTests-Gene Clinics website (National Institutes for Health Gene Tests database 2006). Another important reference source is Wald and Leck's textbook *Antenatal and neonatal screening* (Wald and Leck 2000).

Summary points

In this book we focus on screening programmes aimed at risk reduction for the screened individual, based on sound evidence and delivered to pre-agreed policy and standards.

We take screening to mean the testing of people without signs or symptoms, with the aim of reducing their future risk or giving them information about risk.

Screening tests are like a sieving process, dividing people into higher and lower risk groups, but they do not usually give certainty.

A screening programme is a system incorporating all necessary steps from identifying the eligible population through to delivering interventions and supporting individuals who suffer adverse effects.

Screening will bring more benefit than harm when it is based on sound evidence relating to programme outcomes, and when it is delivered as a quality-assured programme.

Tests and inquiries once signs or symptoms are present are not screening.

Insurance medicals, employment checks, safety checks, infection control tests, epidemiological surveys, and fitness and lifestyle checks have some similarities to screening but they fall outside the definition that we are using in this book.

Thinking at the level of the individual points to the conclusion that any screening could bring a chance of benefit, whereas population thinking weighs up the magnitude of harm and benefit for the population.

Genetic screening is the testing for inherited or heritable disorders, in people without signs or symptoms or known genetic susceptibility. The principles that apply to all screening apply equally to genetic screening.

The special feature of genetic testing is that it can yield information that affects other family members, who did not themselves have a test or give informed consent to the information being uncovered.

Test yourself

Question one

Look at the following list of tests. For each test, think about why it is being done, and try and decide whether it fits our definition of screening, and whether it is being delivered as a programme.

So the first thing to ask yourself is—does it involve a test in a healthy person with the aim of future risk reduction for the condition being tested for, or for information giving that benefits that individual?

For the scenarios that you think are screening, you then need to ask yourself a second question—is the screening being delivered as part of a quality-assured screening programme? You will probably also find yourself asking whether there is sound evidence that the screening does more good than harm at affordable cost, but the information you are supplied with does not enable you to say.

(a) A woman age 50 having an exercise electrocardiogram (ECG or heart trace, also known as the stress test) as part of a 'well person body check' at a private screening clinic.

(b) A man age 55 having a resting electrocardiogram (heart trace) ordered by the anaesthetist, prior to undergoing hernia repair under general anaesthetic.

(c) A man age 20 having a heaf test (a test for presence of tuberculosis infection) because he shares a flat with someone just diagnosed with pulmonary tuberculosis.

(d) A man age 60 having a chest X-ray because he has been coughing up blood.

(e) A man age 50 having a prostate-specific antigen blood test because his friend at the golf club has just been diagnosed with prostate cancer.

(f) A woman age 75 attending a breast screening programme for routine mammography because she thinks it is a good idea to continue with three yearly mammograms, even though regular invitations are only issued up to the age of 71.

(g) A man age 48 having a liver function test before commencing drug treatment that carries a risk of liver toxicity.

(h) A man age 30 having a vision test in order to renew his Heavy Goods Vehicle driver's licence.

(i) A man age 53 having lower bowel endoscopy because he has a rare skin condition that is associated with bowel cancer.

Question two

Think of some different screening programmes that are in existence or that are being planned or researched (the examples shown in the answers are aortic aneurysm screening, congenital hypothyroid screening, sight-threatening diabetic retinopathy screening and cervical screening, so you might like to use these). For each one, see if you can write down the answers to the following questions:

(a) What is the eligible population?

(b) What is the 'sieve', i.e. the screening test or tests?

(c) What is the 'sort', i.e. the diagnostic test or tests?

(d) What is the intervention that is offered?

(e) What is the purpose of the screening, i.e. the adverse outcome that it aims to reduce, or the information that it aims to give and why?

Chapter 3

What screening does

The aim of the chapter

The aim of this chapter is to give you a deeper understanding of screening.

As far as Gould was concerned in 1900 (see Chapter 1, p. 3), the most important question concerning screening was:

- 'Why are we not doing it?'

When Wilson, Holland and others assessed screening in the 1960s (see Chapter 1, p. 10), they asked sophisticated questions about benefit and harm, but at that time this represented too great a change in general thinking. So the question became:

- 'How do we tell if it succeeds in reducing risk?'

This has served us well as a driving force for better evaluation, but it ignores the need also to assess harmful consequences. It has led us into the trap of talking about screening as though a simple dichotomy exists, either 'it works' or 'it doesn't work', all or nothing. Growing experience with organized screening programmes has revealed that we need a more sophisticated question:

- 'What are all the consequences?'

Understanding the range and likelihood of different consequences is important both for decisions about overall policy and for decisions by individuals about whether to participate. Whether any given consequence is seen as 'good' or 'bad' will vary from person to person, so it is important to use neutral and objective terms to describe the outcomes of screening.

Measuring all the consequences of screening is not easy, but it is possible. All too often in the past attempts were made to derive evidence when there was no proper control group for comparison. This is fraught with difficulty. Even where you do have a control group, the tendency up until now has been to measure only the desired outcomes in a research trial, leaving concerns about harms to surface once the screening programme is in place.

In this chapter, we work through the range of different consequences that screening brings. Different observers see some consequences more starkly than others depending on their viewpoint. For example, the family doctor supporting the bereaved relatives of a man who dies from elective repair of a screen-detected aortic aneurysm has a different perspective from the statistician who only analyses data about the benefit. Many disagreements about screening arise purely because different people are looking at different bits of the same thing. Ideally we have to get to a stage where everyone recognizes the complete overview.

Putting people through the screening system

A sieve is only a sieve

In the last chapter we talked about screening tests being like sieves; here is the flow diagram again, but this time it only shows the people who have positive test results (Fig. 3.1).

The steps in a screening process are as follows:

- We identify and invite a subgroup of the whole population who we think are most likely to benefit, for example women over 50 years of age or newborn infants between 2 and 7 days old. We call them the eligible population. They may be individually invited for screening, or there may be general publicity and encouragement to attend, or they may be offered screening if and when they happen to attend medical services for a different reason.

- Those who accept are screened, or poured into the sieve.

- Some, the test positive group, are separated out by the sieving process. They have some degree of abnormality on their test and proceed to the sorting process that looks at them in more detail. Occasionally there is no sorting phase and intervention is offered on the basis of the first test result. For example, a urine test that detects evidence of chlamydia infection may be used in symptomless young people with the aim of reducing complications from chlamydia infection. Antibiotic treatment is given on the basis of

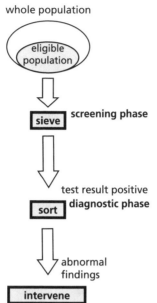

Fig. 3.1 Screening flow diagram for positive tests.

the screening test alone, even though a positive result does not give complete certainty that chlamydia infection is present.

◆ For the moment, the diagram omits the categories not referred for sorting, and not referred for intervention. In practice, many screening tests do not categorize the screened population into only 'screen-positive' and 'screen-negative'. In many programmes there is a third 'in between' category where a repeat test or tests is recommended. We also need to remember that for those who test negative there will always be some who then go on to develop the disease, so we cannot give them complete reassurance that they are at 'no risk'. We will return to these parts of the diagram very soon.

We will now look at where problems can occur along the pathway.

There are problems relating to the tests

No sieve is perfect: the occasional hole may be bigger than it should be, and occasionally a grain of the sieved material may be an odd shape or unusually small. No test is perfect either. The screen-positive group never contains all the cases, and always contains some non-cases. To give an actual example, let us look at antenatal screening for Down's syndrome (National Screening Committee 2003). Several tests, and combinations of tests, are used for Down's screening. These involve biochemical tests on a blood sample from the mother, ultrasound scanning to measure the thickness of tissue and fluid at the back of the baby's neck, and mother's age, which is combined with these measurements to derive a numerical risk of the baby being affected. Even when the screening is performed to a high standard, most of the mothers who screen positive (i.e. they have a high risk score) and who are then offered diagnostic testing do not have Down's babies. So the sieve catches more mothers than just those affected. Also, a tiny minority of the mothers who screen negative (i.e. they have a low risk score) and who do not have diagnostic testing do have a Down's baby. So the sieve lets through some of the cases, and these do not get detected. To put this into numbers, roughly speaking for every 41 mothers who screen positive, one has a Down's baby and 40 do not. For every four screened women with a Down's baby, roughly three will be in the screen-positive group and one will be in the screen-negative group.

There are problems relating to the subjects

The sifted material also presents problems by not always being as distinctly separable as we would wish; thus the rice sieve retains small stones that are of similar size to rice. With human screening, this problem is common because there is seldom a categorical difference between definite normality and definite disease. Rice and stones are completely different from one another, but with human screening we are looking at continuously distributed variables and trying to predict what will happen in the future. Within cervical screening, for example, there are now numerous gradations of cell change categorized by the screening examination, and they are a relatively common finding (Raffle *et al*. 2003). In the 1940s when Papanicolou first advocated cytology screening, the expectation was that only a tiny percentage of women would have clearly abnormal cervical cells, and all others would be normal. The screening concept was based on the logic that because women with cancer were observed to have cancer cells in vaginal samples, then it must follow that if healthy women have abnormal cells then they too will get cancer. The logical flaw is equivalent to arguing that all dogs have four legs therefore anything with four legs is a dog. However, in the 1940s there was no reason to doubt that case definitions based on observation of disease would not hold true when applied to apparent pathology in healthy people. Papanicolou would have been astonished to learn that by the 1990s in the USA the follow-up for women with a grade of abnormal cells on their screening test result known as 'atypical squamous cells of uncertain significance' (ASCUS) would be costing billions of dollars each year.

The sorting can still leave uncertainty

The people who have positive test results on screening (the sieve) are then offered investigations to see if they have the disease, or risk marker, that the screening system is designed to detect. (Although occasionally, as we have explained above, an intervention is offered on the basis of the screening result alone.)

- ◆ If these investigations show abnormality, the person is offered intervention.

- ◆ If the investigations find no abnormality, the person is given some reassurance, but this cannot be complete reassurance, because some who have negative investigations turn out to have the disease, or to develop it soon after they are given a negative result.

- ◆ Often the process of screening and investigating uncovers new categories of borderline disease.

Box 3.1 The polyp puzzle

Screening to reduce deaths from bowel cancer originally aimed to find localized malignant tumours, but once it began, large numbers of people were found to have intestinal polyps. Once pathologists began to examine tissue from these polyps they ran into problems over definitions, nomenclature and gradations of risk. Should these people be put in the category of negative, i.e. normal investigation result? Or should they have their polyps removed and should they be told that they are at higher risk of cancer and

> **Box 3.1 The polyp puzzle** *(cont.)*
>
> need regular colonoscopy? Even after two randomized controlled trials, one in Denmark and one in England (Kronberg *et al.* 1996; Hardcastle *et al.* 1996; Scholefield *et al.* 2002), and a 3 year pilot study of bowel screening in England and Scotland, this question is still not resolved. The evaluation report of the pilot programmes recommends that the pathological classifications still need to be resolved (UKCRC Screening pilot evaluation team 2003). This reflects the huge uncertainty that exists in relation to so-called 'pre-cancerous' conditions, now that we know that in most (but not all) people these tissue changes never give rise to ill health.

Therefore, often our diagram ends up like Fig. 3.2 (see p. 65).

Unless the need for minimizing harm is kept as an explicit objective, it is possible for screening to put large numbers of healthy subjects into a state of uncertainty, and for substantial overtreatment to occur. The fact that some cases are inevitably undetectable is seldom appreciated, and the tendency to use words such as 'missed' or 'screening failures' to describe undetectable cases leads to a perception that mistakes have been made. This provokes a natural reaction among screening staff to 'play safe' and categorize more results as positive or uncertain, and fewer as negative. Subjects with borderline results may end up attending for repeat tests over the course of many years, causing substantial impact on their sense of well-being. One of the purposes of clear policy rules, and measurable standards, is to enable everyone working as part of a screening programme collectively to 'hold their nerve' so that the problem of labelling more and more subjects as abnormal in order to play safe does not get out of control.

There are problems relating to the interventions

Once people have been sieved, sorted and found to have risk markers or symptomless pathological change, they are then offered intervention. Unfortunately, most interventions in healthcare bring the possibility of side effects. Often in screening you are offering interventions

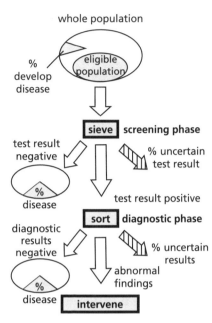

Fig. 3.2 Screening flow diagram with uncertainties and undetected cases.

to a group of people who are extremely worried that they will develop the condition you are trying to prevent, but in truth there is no certainty. It is therefore important to be able to offer effective interventions that are relatively non-invasive and low risk. In the 1960s, young women who wanted to have children in the future were faced with the drastic prospect of hysterectomy for screen-detected 'carcinoma *in situ*' of the cervix. This prompted the development of less invasive treatments that could preserve fertility. These involve local excision and local tissue destruction using laser or heat (diathermy) or cold (cold coagulation).

There are problems relating to the outcome of the intervention

The ordinary man or woman in the street is likely to assume that all the people who receive an intervention have had their health dramatically improved as a result. However, some of those treated would never have developed any problem in relation to the disease being screened for. So their treatment has been pointless. Some would have had a

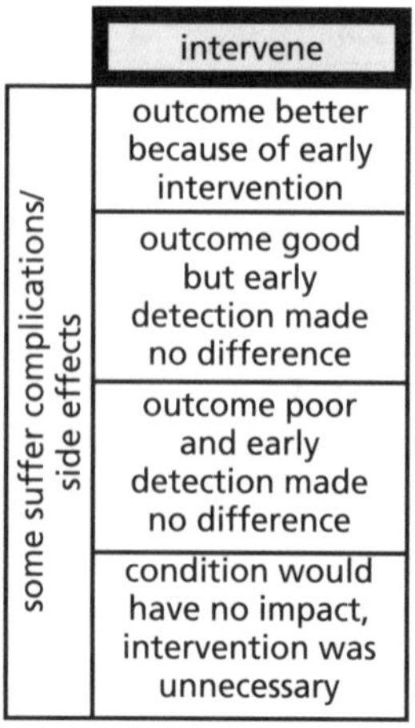

	intervene
some suffer complications/ side effects	outcome better because of early intervention
	outcome good but early detection made no difference
	outcome poor and early detection made no difference
	condition would have no impact, intervention was unnecessary

Fig. 3.3 Outcomes from intervention.

good outcome from treatment even if their disease had been left to present at a symptomatic stage. So their outcome is good, but has been unaltered by the early detection. Some do not do well, even though they have been picked up on screening. In our diagram, we need to add these four subdivisions (Fig. 3.3) within the group that receives intervention. In all four sections, there is the risk of complications or side effects from the treatment.

The concepts of programme sensitivity and specificity

We want our screening process (sieving and sorting) to separate out a group containing as many as possible of those destined to develop the condition that we want to ameliorate. Doing well on this measure is known as having high sensitivity, or in other words having few undetected cases or having a high detection rate. In practice, the term 'sensitivity' applies to the performance of an individual test (see Chapter 4, p. 114), but the concept of sensitivity also applies to the programme and is dependent on the sensitivies at each individual stage. The overall impact on reducing disease in the population is obviously greatest if as many as possible of the future cases have been 'caught' in our group that is offered intervention.

Box 3.2 Maximum benefit

To maximize the benefit we want:

◆ High uptake

◆ High sensitivity/detection rate for both the sieving and the sorting

◆ High acceptance rates for intervention.

We also want our screening process (sieving and sorting) to separate out a group with negative results that contains as many as possible of those destined to stay free of the condition during their lifetime. Doing well on this measure is known as having high specificity, or in other words having few false alarms and little overdiagnosis and overtreatment. Again, specificity is computed for an individual test (see Chapter 4, p. 114), but the concept can be applied to the whole programme.

Also, we want to minimize harm by ensuring that people understand what is on offer. If you try and conceal information about limitations and side effects, this only means that the bad news has a more damaging effect when it does emerge. Some people find it very difficult to cope with uncertainty, with repeated investigations and follow-ups, or with developing disease that was not picked up on screening, particularly if they feel that the implied promise of screening was very different from their experience. It is important to give people realistic expectations.

Box 3.3 Minimum harm

To minimize the harm we want:

◆ High specificity/low-false positive rate for both sieving and sorting

◆ Individuals to understand what is on offer and to think carefully about whether participation is right for them.

We can trade maximizing benefit with minimizing harm.

♦ By changing the tests or the thresholds at both screening and diagnostic stages of the programme, we can vary the balance between catching as many future cases as possible and correctly reassuring as many as possible of those destined to remain free of the disease. This is like varying the performance of a sieve by altering the size of the holes. Widening or narrowing the eligible population can also have an effect.

♦ By changing the information we give, we can attract or deter people from attending, and a balance is needed to ensure that people can understand the benefits without overlooking the potential drawbacks.

The popularity paradox

In most screening programmes, some people receive treatment who would never have developed a problem if they had been left unscreened. They do not realize that they are victims of overdiagnosis or overtreatment. This is because everyone with screen-detected abnormality is offered intervention, and even if we know that say 40 have to be treated to prevent one serious outcome, we cannot know who is the one and who are the 39. So any of those treated could have derived major benefit, and most tend to believe that they are the one. We call this the 'popularity paradox'. The greater the overdiagnosis and overtreatment, the more people there are who believe they owe their health or even their life to the programme.

Box 3.4 The popularity paradox

The greater the harm through overdiagnosis and overtreatment from screening, the more people there are who believe they owe their health, or even their life, to the programme.

The pressure to avoid missed cases

In contrast, people realize when they are an undetected case because they develop the disease despite the fact that they attended for screening.

Many feel extremely angry and let down because they believed, wrongly, that a negative screening result was a guarantee.

This means that public and media pressure tends to drive increases in sensitivity even at the cost of more overtreatment as a consequence. Policy and practice often drift, or are explicitly changed, in an attempt to bolster public confidence and to avoid the headline news stories and legal action that accompany the cases not picked up by screening.

It is possible to counter this by setting standards designed to minimize false positives and by accepting, and explaining, the inevitability of undetected cases. Standards in the UK breast screening programme, for example, require that the percentage of women recalled for assessment (the sort) following mammography (the sieve) has to be less than 7 per cent and the rate of benign biopsies has to be less than 2 per 1000 screens (this is the standard applied to first attendances which are known as 'incidence' screens) (NHS Breast Screening Programme 2005). The existence of such controls to guard against overinvestigation and overdiagnosis varies from programme to programme internationally, and cumulative false-positive rates for mammography screening vary substantially from country to country, with the highest cumulative false-positive rates being in the USA (Christiansen *et al.* 2000; Elmore *et al.* 2003; Smith-Bindman *et al.* 2003). Adherence to standards such as those quoted above, together with access to the woman's previous films at the time of reading, making it easier to judge any change on appearance (this is possible where screening is organized as a programme, but difficult if providers just offer tests), are the likely reasons for the lower false-positive rates in certain countries. Ductal carcinoma *in situ* (DCIS) a condition where the cells in the breast tissue have the appearance of cancer cells but are not appearing to behave invasively, also has higher detection rates in the USA (Ernster *et al.* 1996). Many women faced with the knowledge that they have DCIS choose to have mastectomy, but most of them would not go on to develop cancer in their lifetime. The result is unnecessary intervention and some harmful side effects.

So the pressure to avoid missed cases tends to lead to harm from overinvestigation, overdiagnosis and overtreatment. This can be counteracted to some extent by setting standards for maximum positive rates, recall rates and intervention rates.

The experience for those being screened

The people in the two by two table

Traditionally the performance of a test is summarized as a two by two table, with the test result down the side, the truth or some best proxy for it along the top, and letters in the boxes so that you can show the formulae for sensitivity and specificity (see Chapter 4, p. 114).

For the people being screened, the test is only the first step, and in thinking through their experience we need to take account of what happens subsequently.

We can use the two by two table to show what people typically experience when the initial screening test (the sieving phase) divides them into the different groups—true and false positive, and true and false negative.

Once we do this, we see that the two by two table is too simple because of the overdiagnosis of inconsequential disease that occurs with screening. The true positives category therefore needs to be subdivided into those destined to develop serious disease, and those not. The international group writing for the series of evidence-based guides published in the *Journal of the American Medical Association* achieved this using a three by two table, and subdividing the categories as true and 'true', false and 'false' (Barratt *et al.* 1999).

In Table 3.1 we illustrate this using the example of three yearly mammography screening for reducing deaths from breast cancer, and considering a single screening round. There are six boxes in this table:

Table 3.1 The three by two table for screening

		The Truth		
		Breast pathology that would become symptomatic breast cancer	Breast pathology that would have remained latent	No breast pathology and not destined to develop symptomatic disease before next routine screen
The Test (mammography)	Positive	True positive	'True' positives	False positives
	Negative	False negatives	'False' negatives	True negatives

The true positives are those who have an abnormal (positive) mammogram, and who have breast cancer that will in the future develop into significant disease if left untreated.

- Initially they feel devastated, having gone for their routine test hoping for the all-clear but instead learning that they have a life-threatening disease.

- Further investigation follows, then treatment, and most do well. For some, their good outcome would have been the same had they not had screening, but these women are indistinguishable from those where screening has made the all-important difference. All are likely to feel thankful they went for the screening and that they owe their lives to the programme.

- Some have progressive, eventually fatal disease despite treatment and despite being picked up on screening. They may feel thankful that screening gave them the best chance of cure. Alternatively, they may feel let down because for them screening did not fulfil its apparent promise.

The 'true' positives are women who have an abnormal mammogram, and who have breast cancer that would not have developed into significant disease during the woman's lifetime. Several different words are used to describe this phenomenon. Gilbert Welch from the Dartmouth Medical School in the USA uses the term pseudodisease in his wonderfully clear description of the overdiagnosis and overtreatment problems in cancer screening (Welch 2004). Another frequently used term is latent disease, and a third term is inconsequential disease. Evidence that the treatment of latent cases is a significant problem in breast screening has been mounting for the last 20 years but as yet women are not informed about it. The case study below on overdiagnosis in breast screening explains the evidence.

- The 'true' positive women feel exactly the same as the true positives, are managed in the same way and are indistinguishable from them because all have to be offered treatment just in case. It is not possible to tell these women with latent disease from those whose disease would progress. Indeed the factors that make the difference may relate to genetic attributes or to environmental insults that have not happened yet for that woman.

- Almost all the women in this group are likely to feel thankful they went for the screening and that they owe their lives to the programme, even though some suffer harm from the treatment that they did not actually need.

- A few well informed women are shocked to discover the uncertainties associated with a screen detected diagnosis, particularly if they have DCIS, and they may question whether treatment is needed if they do not have invasive cancer. The DCIS problem is not yet mentioned in the information materials available to women considering screening in the UK. Christine Johnson, patient representative on the Board of one regional NHS cancer organization, described her efforts to find reliable information about DCIS as like trying to 'uncover a closely guarded state secret' (Johnson 2004). Hazel Thornton, who had DCIS detected on screening and chose to decline treatment, highlights the General Medical Council's advice that responsible citizens need adequate information to give consent for screening, and argues 'so, too, do those angry women whose bodies and lives, and the lives of their families, have been damaged by this zealous trawling to find breast cancer early' (Thornton 1999).

Case 3.1 Case study—overdiagnosis in breast cancer screening

There are two main sources of evidence that show for certain that overdiagnosis is a problem.

- First there are post-mortem studies showing that the prevalence of undiagnosed *in situ* and invasive breast histopathological lesions far exceeds the level that can be explained by known incidence (Nielsen 1989; Welch and Black 1997), and that the harder pathologists look the more cases are found. Welch and Black use the term 'reservoir' of disease, and conclude that this 'has important implications for what it means to have disease'.

Case 3.1 Case study—overdiagnosis in breast cancer screening *(cont.)*

♦ Secondly there is the finding that screen-detected cumulative incidence of breast cancer exceeds the incidence prior to screening, and in unscreened age-matched control groups and non-screened age bands (Zahl *et al.* 2004; Møller *et al.* 2005; Zackrisson *et al.* 2006). If there were no overdiagnosis then this would not happen.

This important problem was featured in 2006 in a collection of articles and correspondence in the *British Medical Journal* (Baum 2006; Gøtzsche 2006; Irwig *et al.* 2006; Møller and Davies 2006; Thornton 2006; Welch *et al.* 2006; Zahl and Maehlen 2006).

♦ Overall the conclusions were that for each one woman who has her life prolonged by mammography screening, at least two women (but probably more) have treatment with breast removal, cancer drugs and radiotherapy for cancers that would have remained latent and never caused a problem in their lifetimes.

♦ At least one-quarter, and possibly one-third of the breast cancer cases picked up on screening would remain unknown were it not for screening, and would never cause a problem.

Later in 2006 an update of the Cochrane review of breast cancer screening (Gøtzsche and Nielsen 2006) summarized the overdiagnosis harm as follows:

> for every 2000 women invited for screening throughout ten years, one will have her life prolonged. In addition, ten healthy women, who would not have been diagnosed if there had not been screening, will be diagnosed as breast cancer patients and will be treated unnecessarily.

So for every 200 women screened during 10 years, one is a 'true' positive (as defined in our three by two table) and is subjected to cancer treatment that she does not need.

The Cochrane reviewers concluded, as many others have done, that women invited for screening should be fully informed of both benefits and harms. This is serious stuff and is of great concern to many people involved in delivering screening. Outside of the scientific community though, the idea that healthy women are being harmed by mastectomy, radiotherapy and chemotherapy that they do not need is still met with disbelief and denial.

The false positives are women who have an abnormal mammogram but who do not have breast cancer.

- Initially they feel just as fearful as the true positives but, once they return for their assessment (the sorting process), which includes ultrasound and fine needle aspiration cytology or core biopsy, they are then given the all clear.

- These women suffer a temporary false alarm. How they feel about it varies. Most find it worrying but still rate screening as a positive event and return for subsequent screens. A few feel that mistakes must have been made, particularly if they were not aware that one in every 10 women is recalled yet few have cancer.

- A few are left with lasting fears that maybe the screen was right and the sorting process missed something. If enough women are screened, then sooner or later this will turn out to be true for someone.

The false negatives are those who have breast cancer that will in the future develop into significant disease if left untreated, but who have a negative result on screening, or in other words their mammogram report is normal.

- These women feel relieved and reassured.

- Then, at some stage during the 3 years before their next routine test, they are diagnosed clinically with breast cancer.

- These women are likely to feel let down by screening, although if they are well informed they will know that undetected cases are an inevitable event in all screening programmes.

- Some may feel that the outcome of their cancer will have been adversely affected if they, or their doctor, delayed seeking investigation for signs or symptoms because of false reassurance from their negative screening result.

- One reason for normal mammography followed by clinical diagnosis is that a true 'interval' cancer occurred. The breast cancer was not there at the time of the screen, but arose thereafter.

- A second reason is that the breast cancer does not show on mammography. About 7 per cent of breast cancers do not show up on X-ray.

◆ A third reason is that the shadow caused by the cancer was indistinguishable from the numerous shadows in a normal breast. Now that the cancer has grown, one can look back at the past film and say 'there it was', but without the benefit of hindsight a competent observer reports the film as negative.

◆ A fourth reason is that the film reader overlooked the abnormality. On looking back at the film there is a visible abnormal shadow. All film readers should be trained, undergo regular proficiency tests, have their film reading performance figures regularly checked and should follow rules about taking breaks and about their working environment in order to reduce risk of distraction and attention fatigue. Even film readers who meet all these quality standards have occasional undetected cases. It is a phenomenon of the human brain that temporary attention lapses are inevitable, and this applies whether it is cancer screening, or visual checking of electronic circuits in aircraft assembly, or scrutiny of radar screens to detect enemy aircraft. We try and overcome this in breast screening by double reading—so that two independent observers screen every mammogram. Even this cannot eliminate all the missed cases. It could even mean that the observers, knowing there is double reading, are less vigilant.

The 'false' negatives are women who have latent disease but a normal mammogram.

◆ They feel relieved and reassured.

◆ They are better off not being picked up on screening because they avoid the fear and anxiety of being diagnosed and pointlessly treated for breast cancer, and they avoid any side effects from investigations and treatment.

The true negatives are women who do not have breast cancer and who have a normal mammogram.

◆ They feel relieved and reassured.

◆ They are likely to feel that their normal result puts them at far lower risk than they were before their test (Black *et al.* 1995). In fact the absolute difference is very slight. Based on the Swedish trial data, a woman who had just had a negative mammogram could be 99.8 per cent confident that she would not be diagnosed with breast cancer by the time her next screen was due. If she had not attended, then she could be 99.4 per cent confident of not being diagnosed with breast cancer during the same interval. So the absolute difference in risk between a woman who has not had a screen, and the same woman once she has had a negative screen, is very small (Schmidt 1990).

What do we mean by 'true'

You could argue that our 'true' positives are not any kind of true positive, they are actually false positives because the person is not destined to develop life-impacting disease. This takes us back to Wittgenstein and the need to pay attention to words and their meaning. We suspect that the terms true positive and false positive cause more confusion than clarity because they mean different things to different people. For this reason we try to avoid using these terms wherever possible, and we have not used them in our flowchart. In the language of screening, a true positive is one that fits the case definition for the condition being screened for. The case definition for screen-detected breast cancer relates to the pathological changes visible in a tissue specimen and judged by a trained and competent pathologist. Pathologists cannot foretell the future, they can only describe what they see. Saying that someone is a true case is not the same as saying that they will definitely suffer life-impacting disease if left untreated, although this distinction would not be at all clear to the ordinary person.

The system and its outcomes

As a final exercise, we just need to check how this three by two table relates back to our screening flow diagram.

- The true positives are represented by three sections of the intervention group; those who have benefit, those who would have had a good outcome anyway, and those who have poor outcome despite being picked up and treated.

- The 'true' positives are represented by the fourth section in the intervention group showing those with unnecessary intervention.

- The false positives, who suffer a false alarm on the initial screening process but then have normal findings on investigation, are the lower circle of reassured individuals. There is a subset of this group that will develop disease, because some will develop interval disease. Some will have had abnormality that was not picked up even on investigation.

♦ The false negatives are the 'develop disease' subset of the upper circle of reassured individuals, who tested normal on screening but later turned out to develop the disease. As we explained in the section above, there are different reasons for false negatives; some are interval cases and some are not picked up because of limitations of the test.

♦ The true negatives, and the 'false' negatives, are the remainder of the upper circle of reassured individuals.

Disease in people not invited

Another important fact is that people outside the eligible population will get the disease. This is represented by the section we have added within the whole population, and it finally completes our diagram (Fig. 3.4).

An example is that women under 50 (the lower age limit for mammography screening) do get breast cancer. If the public are led to believe that screening is simple, prevents all disease in those screened and pays for itself, then the fact that anyone at risk is excluded from the invited population just does not make sense. Such a simple and cost-saving approach must surely be made available to anyone at risk. This illustrates the problem we will always face unless and until clear information about the consequences of screening becomes readily accessible, enabling public understanding of screening to improve.

Can't make your mind up categories

We hope that by now it is clear that a major headache for those running screening is that it is difficult to force clinicians, pathologists, radiologists, geneticists, clinical chemists, or whoever, to stick with only two outcomes at both the screening stage and the sorting stage. Always people want an extra category in between reassurance or investigation, or in between reassurance or intervention. However, the reality is that even a normal test result on screening can never give a guarantee.

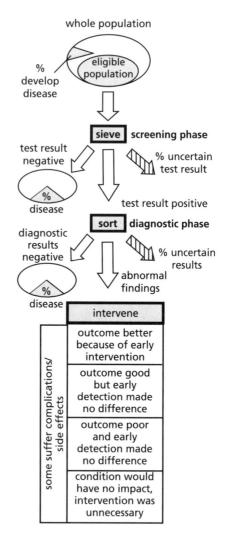

Fig. 3.4 The screening process.

The consequence of creating additional uncertain categories for whom repeated tests and follow-up are recommended is that much uncertainty is created for those undergoing screening and, paradoxically, more and more resources end up being devoted to groups at very low risk, by testing them repeatedly and tracking them all over the country when they change name, address or family doctor. A great deal of harm is caused when clinicians cannot or will not make their minds up concerning the results of screening examinations.

Finding other things

If you talk to people doing screening and ask them what they are actually looking for, you will get very different answers. Some believe the screening task to be solely about finding things that fit your case definition for that screening programme. Your evidence only relates to that condition and your commitment is that you are offering participation in a programme known to reduce risk for that condition. Other people give a very different answer, and feel they are looking for anything at all that is not entirely normal. For example, some pathologists report infection that they see in cervical cytology screening samples, whereas others do not because if an infection is clinically significant it will be diagnosed and treated. If it is not significant, and most of them are not, then why report it. These reports of infection cause confusion and distress for the women, and dilemmas for their family doctors.

Apparent abnormalities are actually incredibly common in healthy people and most are completely harmless. Transient self-limiting processes cause them—infections, benign cysts, cellular change that is repaired—so in effect although they look abnormal most of these changes are part and parcel of the hidden processes going on in normal healthy human beings. This problem becomes ever more significant as modern imaging techniques become so powerful they show up every tiny cyst. For example, conventional colonoscopy, where the colon is examined using a fibreoptic tube, can now be replaced by virtual colonoscopy using CT scanning. For those who can afford it, this is used as a screening method for reducing risk of bowel cancer in the USA. One effect of this is that shadows and bumps in other organs show up, and healthy people then need highly invasive further investigations in order to check whether these findings are innocent or not.

Who is helped and who is harmed?

After working through the table and the diagram, you may have concluded that this question has a slightly fuzzy answer. To the public health purist, the only people genuinely helped are those who avoid death or serious disease as a direct result of early detection and early intervention. Everyone else would do just as well, or would be better off, if they had not participated in the screening. This is very different though from how screening appears to the individual participant or to the clinician. As we said at the start of the chapter, it all depends on your viewing point. Population and individual perspectives diverge substantially when it comes to the matters of overtreatment, the value of reassurance and the problem of medicalizing normal life.

Does overtreatment matter if individuals are happy?

By and large everyone who has screen-detected abnormality feels thankful for the screening programme. The clinicians treating them often believe that they have cured them all. It is only indirectly, from looking at population numbers and at results from controlled trials, that we know we are only improving the health outcome for a minority of those with screen-detected disease.

This is a difficult problem for public health practitioners because our 'patient' is the population, so the principle in the Hippocratic oath of 'first do no harm' is contravened in programmes that do more harm than good.

However, for the individual, the concept of harm from screening is counterintuitive. Take for example Diana Ward's excellent book of breast cancer patients' stories (Ward 1996). Each chapter is about a different person, and one is of a woman whose entire life is dominated by severe intractable pain following prophylactic mastectomy and failed reconstructive surgery for carcinoma *in situ*. The distinct possibility that this pre-cancerous condition would never have caused her a problem and that her suffering is entirely a medically induced harm never even crosses the patient's mind, or if it has then she has quickly dismissed it.

How valuable is reassurance?

Many people attending for screening say that they have come because they want the reassurance of a negative test. We have even heard politicians, senior civil servants and clinicians say that reassurance of healthy people is a, perhaps even the, legitimate aim of screening. Our own view is that the reassurance given by screening is largely an illusion (for mammography an absolute difference in risk of 4 per 1000, see p. 76), that it leads to harm if symptoms are ignored and that it leads to medicalization. By this we mean the undermining of people's confidence in their own health, the undermining of primary prevention as the means of safeguarding health, the creation of a myth that technological tests are more reliable than they truly are and the creation of dependence on regular medical tests. As Peter Gøtzsche, head of the Nordic Cochrane Centre puts it 'Do we wish to turn the world's healthy citizens into fearful patients-to-be?' (Gøtzsche 1997). Another major problem with screening only to provide reassurance is the opportunity cost. It ties up a lot of healthcare resources that are then unavailable for caring for ill people.

A populist consumerist view would be that our arguments about medicalization are just highbrow paternalism and if people want screening for reassurance they should have it. But even so, we still come back to 'well alright but who pays and how'.

Summary points

For participants offered screening, and for people outside the eligible group, the delivery of screening changes their experience in diverse ways. This is summarized by the final version of the screening flowchart shown in Fig. 3.4.

Almost all screening uncovers inconsequential disease and uncovers categories of abnormality for which the prognosis is unknown.

There is always a trade-off between sensitivity and specificity. High sensitivity means catching as many of the cases as possible. It means you have more false alarms, overdiagnosis and overtreatment, but fewer undetected cases. High specificity means giving negative results to as many as possible of the people without the condition. It means you have more undetected cases but have fewer false alarms, overdiagnosis and overtreatment.

Participants and clinicians can find it very hard to accept that some people develop the disease despite participation in screening.

> **Summary points** *(cont.)*
>
> This tends to make people err on the side of caution, with the result that the programme becomes more sensitive but with very poor specificity. Robust policy and performance standards are needed to prevent this.
>
> Overdiagnosis and overtreatment create a paradoxical popularity because each individual justifies their experience by believing that they have had a dramatic benefit.
>
> Many disagreements about screening are because different people focus exclusively on only one or two consequences, and fail to acknowledge the complete picture.

Test yourself

Question one

In this question we use screening for abdominal aortic aneurysm as the example.

An abdominal aortic aneurysm is an abnormal enlargement of the major artery carrying blood from the heart to the lower limbs. Aneurysms can rupture, sometimes resulting in slow leakage of blood but sometimes catastrophically. Emergency surgery to repair the aorta may save some people, particularly if the leak is slow, but most sudden ruptures lead to death. It is possible to screen for aneurysms using ultrasound examination to measure the diameter of the abdominal aorta, and then surgically to repair large aneurysms found as a result. The definition of 'large' 'medium' and 'small' is inevitably arbitrary, and the size is only an indicator of risk, as some large aneurysms never rupture and some small ones do. A size of 50–55 mm diameter is regarded as large enough to warrant elective surgical repair. The eligible group for screening is usually defined on the basis of risk and fitness for surgery. Predominantly this means men aged over 60 and under 75, particularly if they have risk factors for vascular disease. CT scanning may be used as a diagnostic procedure following the ultrasound screen, but it is feasible to decide on intervention on the basis of the ultrasound alone.

See if you can map out all the possible consequences for participants undergoing abdominal aortic aneurysm screening using the format of the flowchart in Fig. 3.4. Be sure to include descriptions for each of the four different categories within the group that receives intervention.

Question two

Imagine you have just undergone screening for aortic aneurysm. You have been told that you do have an aneurysm but that it's size is below the threshold where surgical repair would be recommended. You are advised to have a repeat ultrasound examination at some time in the future to see if the size has changed. Jot down:

- how you think you would feel immediately after you were given the news
- how you think you would feel 3 months later
- how you think you would feel immediately before your 6 months ultrasound
- what information you would want to have been given before you had made your initial decision to accept the first screening ultrasound examination.

Question three

You are advising a national health department on the setting up of a screening programme for abdominal aortic aneurysm. The officials want to consider a range of options to help them decide what balance to strike between the two extremes of either:

(A) a programme that would have a minimum of undetected cases, in other words a very sensitive programme, or

(B) a programme that would have a minimum of overdiagnosis and overintervention, in other words a very specific programme.

Below is a list of features. Categorize each feature according to whether it belongs to A (sensitive programme, minimum undetected) or B (specific programme, minimum overdiagnosis and overtreatment).

(a) Wide eligibility, for example all men age 55–84, and all women age 60–84 with specified risk factors.

(b) Large diameter as the cut-off for initiating ultrasound monitoring, say 40 mm.

(c) Regular screening examinations, say three yearly.

(d) Low threshold for offering surgery, for example 40 mm, or 30 mm if they are showing any signs of increasing in size.

(e) Narrow eligibility covering only men age 60 or over and with risk factors.

(f) Selective policy for offering surgical repair, for example only aneurysms 55 mm or more in people who are fit for surgery.

(g) Small diameter as the cut-off for initiating ultrasound monitoring, say 30 mm.

(h) Once-only screening examination.

(i) Frequent ultrasound monitoring, say three monthly initially, then six monthly for aneurysms that appear to be staying stable, and continue indefinitely.

(j) Selective ultrasound monitoring, for example one ultrasound at a year in people with an aneurysm below 40—55 mm then no further examinations unless there has been substantial increase in size from the previous examination.

Question four

Jot down the main advantages and disadvantages for each of the two different approaches to screening considered in question three above.

Chapter 4

Measuring what screening does

The aim of the chapter

The aim of this chapter is to give you an understanding of evidence about screening. It aims for the level needed by a public health practitioner who has to interpret evidence for setting screening policy, or for ensuring high quality service delivery. It does not give the depth of knowledge you would need for designing and running a trial.

At the risk of oversimplifying, we have condensed the subject down to:

- Three main biases
  - Healthy screenee effect
  - Length time effect
  - Lead time effect
- Three main evaluation methods
  - Randomized controlled trials (RCTs)
  - Time trend analyses
  - Case–control studies
- Two additional sources of information
  - Pilot or demonstration projects
  - Modelling
- Test performance
  - Sensitivity and specificity
  - Positive and negative predictive value
  - Receiver operator characteristic curves

- ◆ Summarizing information on all outcomes
  - The numbers in the flow diagram
  - Decision aids.

Three main sources of bias in screening evaluation

> Reading the facts about screening is like the intellectual equivalent of a cold shower.
>
> Martyn (1999)

If all you do is measure health in screened people then you will quickly become convinced that screening reduces risk from all kinds of diseases. This is because the kind of people who come for screening, and the kind of disease that it is easy to find with screening, add up to a highly selected group with regard both to the overall health and longevity of the individuals and to the benign natural course of the uncovered pathology. The combined effect is a very favourable prognosis. Outcomes in screened people will therefore be very good, whether or not screening makes a difference. Three key biases are at work. These biases make it impossible to gain reliable evidence from observational studies, or in other words from studies that lack a proper control group. This is why a well conducted randomized trial is the most reliable way of telling what difference screening makes.

The healthy screenee effect

People who come for screening tend to be healthier than those who do not. This is the finding from numerous studies, one of which is shown in the following case study. The reason seems to be that healthy, well educated, affluent, physically fit, fruit and vegetable eating, non-smokers with long-lived parents are more likely to come and get screened than people on a low income, who have existing health and social problems, are smokers, drinkers, physically inactive, have a poor diet and whose parents died young. The reasons are multiple. Lack of resources, lack of freedom to miss time from work, carer duties and existing poor physical and mental health all play a part. In addition, screening non-attenders by and large tend to be more chaotic, to feel that their poor health is inevitable and nothing they can do will influence it, and to feel reluctant to submit to a test which might simply burden them with yet another health problem. The dilemma for the researcher is that the healthy screenee effect makes it impossible to know (without a proper control group) whether better outcomes in screened individuals are caused by the screening, or whether they are just the result you would expect anyway when observing a self-selected group of healthier people. It also poses real problems with delivering screening, since the highest risk groups are the least likely to come even if you make services highly accessible.

Case 4.1 Case study—the New York Health Insurance Plan trial

A large randomized trial of mammography breast screening took place in New York during the 1960s (Shapiro 1977). Three hundred thousand women were randomized either to be offered screening, or not, and all women were followed-up.

After 5 years, data for deaths **other than breast cancer** showed the following:

- There was no significant difference in death rates from causes excluding breast cancer between the study group that was offered screening and the control group that was not offered screening. The rate was 56.9 per 10 000 in women offered screening, and 57.6 per 10 000 in women not offered screening. This is to be expected, and confirms that randomization has produced comparable groups.

- Within the group offered screening, there were significant differences in non-breast cancer deaths between the accepters and the refusers. The death rate in women who accepted the invitation and attended for screening was only half what it was in women who declined the invitation and did not attend. The figures were 42.4 per 10 000 in women who had screening, and 85.6 per 10 000 in women who did not. The difference was highly statistically significant, which means that it was not likely to be due to chance.

Case 4.1 Case study—the New York Health Insurance Plan trial *(cont.)*

What is the most likely explanation for the lower death rate in women who attended screening?

The two basic possibilities are either:

- the observed difference in death rate is because of inherent differences between the two groups of women, the refusers and the accepters, or

- the observed difference in death rate is a result of the intervention that one group receives but the other does not.

One could argue that attending for the mammography might prompt lifestyle changes because of advice given by the staff, or because the whole process causes women to reflect on their own health. This explanation is completely implausible. For one thing, the death rate from causes other than breast cancer in the entire offered screening group is identical to that in the control group. So the intervention has made no difference to these deaths. In addition, trials that have compared outcomes in groups randomized to receive, or not receive, intensive lifestyle advice have found only small changes in health-related behaviour and no measurable change in deaths (Family Heart Study Group 1994; OXCHECK Study Group 1995).

The only possible explanation is that the significant difference in death rates is due to inherent difference between the self-selected groups. Women who attend for screening tend to be highly educated, with no health or social problems, on a reasonable income and non-smokers. Women who do not attend for screening tend to have no full-time education beyond age 16, many existing health and social problems, be on a low income and are smokers. Any measure of health status will be better in those who attend for screening.

The Health Insurance Plan trial data are illustrating the 'healthy screenee effect'.

Now imagine that we show you a similar difference between screened and unscreened women but for breast cancer deaths, and that we present it as though the unscreened women are a valid comparison group. It would be easy to conclude that the mammography,

> **Case 4.1 Case study—the New York Health Insurance Plan trial** *(cont.)*
>
> rather than the group selection, is the reason for the difference. This conclusion would be completely unreliable. The only valid comparison is between all of the offered screening group including those who accepted and those who did not, and all of the not offered, in other words the control group. This is what the Health Insurance Plan trial was designed for, and the trial did find that breast cancer deaths were less in the group offered screening compared with those not offered screening.

Length time effect

Screening is best at picking up long-lasting non-progressive or slowly progressive pathological conditions. This pulls good prognosis cases into your group of screen-detected cases, and leaves out the poor prognosis rapidly progressive cases that screening has little chance of detecting. This means that the outcome in a group of screen-detected cases is automatically better than the outcome in a group of clinically diagnosed cases whose disease presented with signs or symptoms, even if screening makes absolutely no difference at all to outcome. The two groups—screen-detected cases on the one hand, clinically presenting cases on the other—are not comparable. This is why case definitions are so important, and why screen-detected cases can never be assumed to be directly comparable with clinically detected cases. The following case study, and the diagrams in Fig. 4.1, illustrate the length time effect.

Case 4.2 Case study—screening infants for neuroblastoma

In 1985 in Japan, a nationwide infant screening programme for neuroblastoma began. Neuroblastoma is a form of childhood cancer that tends to have a poor prognosis if it presents above the age of 1, and a more favourable prognosis in infants who present under 1.

Case 4.2 Case study—screening infants for neuroblastoma *(cont.)*

In 1990, an international panel met in Chicago USA to address the question 'Do children benefit from mass screening for neuro-blastoma' (Murphy *et al.* 1991). The panel reviewed data from Japan and elsewhere. The following facts were clear:

- In Japan during the first 3 years of screening, over 337 infants had been diagnosed by screening, 97 per cent of whom were alive following treatment.

- The number of infants presenting above 1 year of age with neuroblastoma in Japan showed no change.

- The death rate from neuroblastoma in Japan appeared to be following a similar pattern to that of countries that were not screening.

- The incidence of neuroblastoma in Japan had increased substantially since the introduction of screening.

The panel was faced with the problem of working out whether infants were benefiting from the screening, but they had no control group data to use for comparison.

- One possibility is that screening is picking up latent cases, which would never have caused symptoms. This inflates the incidence and, because these cases have an excellent prognosis, produces an apparently impressive outcome in the screen-detected group. However, no infants have actually had their outcome improved, least of all those with serious disease.

- The alternative possibility is that Japan was on the brink of an epidemic and screening began just in time to control it. That is why the incidence rises, and although deaths and late presentations stay the same they would have risen were it not for the screening programme.

The panel diplomatically commended the pioneering work of the Japanese, but concluded that:

- Screening was making no difference in serious cases, and was leading to detection of disease that would never have been manifest clinically.

Case 4.2 Case study—screening infants for neuroblastoma *(cont.)*

- The effectiveness of mass screening for neuroblastoma remained unproven, and physicians and the public needed to know this.
- Implementation of neuroblastoma screening could not be recommended.
- Randomized controlled trials needed to be supported.

Following the Chicago report, two randomized controlled trials have been conducted, one in Canada and one in Germany (Schilling *et al.* 2002; Woods *et al.* 2002). These have confirmed that with current techniques for detection and intervention, screening does not reduce mortality, but does result in harm— sometimes fatal harm—from complications of treatment.

The impressive 97 per cent survival in the screen-detected cases in Japan between 1985 and 1988 is an example of the length time effect or length time bias. It looks like a dramatic 'improvement' on the 50–55 per cent 5-year survival rate for neuroblastoma cases in an unscreened population. The explanation is not that more infants have been cured, it is just that the 337 cases include infants whose condition is present for a relatively long time without causing symptoms. These cases are relatively easy to pick up on screening because they exist for a long time (hence the name length time bias). Most of these cases have a good prognosis and in fact some would regress. Also, the 337 cases exclude the worst prognosis cases. These arise and progress in a short space of time and are not easily picked up by screening.

Faced with only the survival rate statistic, and with a popular programme, a strong clinical lobby and the difficulty of explaining length time bias, it can be hard to take the rigorous approach that the Chicago panel stuck to. The fact that they did has saved many children from the complications of futile treatment. At the time of the Chicago meeting, persuasive marketing of neuroblastoma testing, particularly to developing countries, was just starting, and small pilot studies without control groups were looking at feasibility and acceptability of screening. Thanks to the critical scrutiny achieved by the Chicago panel, pilot study results were not misinterpreted as evidence of benefit (Craft *et al.* 1992).

Case 4.2 Case study—screening infants for neuroblastoma *(cont.)*

In Japan, once the trials were reported, a committee was established by the Japanese Ministry of Health, Labour and Welfare to review the national policy. This resulted in a decision to halt the national programme (Tsubono and Hisamichi 2004). From April 2004 in Japan, infant screening for neuroblastoma ceased. This straightforward approach to acting on the evidence might be hard to achieve in some countries, and in Chapter 8 (see p. 232) we look at the sharply contrasting case of the mammography wars in the USA. Several factors were relevant in the Japanese situation (Yoshitaka Tsubono personal communication):

- The media were generally supportive of the Government recommendation. Many screening programmes in Japan had been introduced without prior evidence, and a best-selling book in Japan some 10 years earlier, by a physician, had succeeded in raising public awareness about the pitfalls of cancer screening unless there was proper evidence.

- The test was done by mailing of a filter paper urine test, which parents performed and returned to the public health centres. There was little advertising or promotion of the programme, it just happened. There was therefore fairly low awareness amongst parents of the purpose of the test or of neuroblastoma, and there were no advocacy groups in favour of screening.

This case study shows how the results of observational studies can be totally misleading, because of the phenomenon known as length time effect or length time bias. Figure 4.1 illustrates the concept in diagrammatic form. The figure is in two parts. First we have Fig. 4.1a, which shows the cases in a population of 100 000. There is no screening so the only cases that are apparent are the five clinical cases that progress to having symptoms. Three of these five cases are amenable to cure or control. Two are fatal despite diagnosis and treatment.

There are in addition three cases where a detectable pathological change is present but where progression to symptomatic disease will not occur in the person's lifetime. We have labelled these as inconsequential cases. The terms latent disease or pseudodisease are also used commonly to describe this type of case. These are symptomless cases and will remain latent, and in the absence of screening they remain undiscovered.

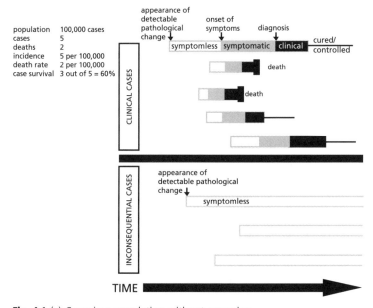

Fig. 4.1 (a) Cases in a population without screening.

The disease statistics without screening are:

◆ Incidence is five cases per 100 000

◆ Death rate is two per 100 000

◆ Case survival is three out of five, or 60 per cent.

Figure 4.1b shows the same population, and illustrates what happens if everyone is screened, on two occasions, to detect the pathological change that exists in symptomless cases. In this theoretical example, the screen is just a test with no subsequent action, as all we are doing is showing what happens to the disease *statistics* because of testing. The duration of the symptomless phase in the most serious cases is very short, so neither of the fatal cases are picked up on screening. These two cases are diagnosed clinically between screens. Two out of the three clinical but non-fatal cases are picked up on screening, and one is diagnosed clinically between screens. The duration of the symptomless phase in the inconsequential cases is long, and all these cases are picked up on screening.

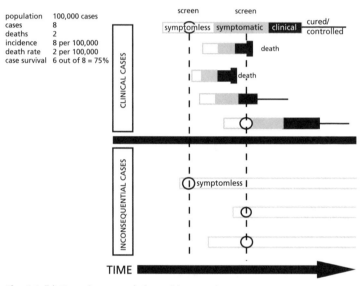

Fig. 4.1 (b) Cases in a population with screening.

The disease statistics with screening are:

◆ Incidence is eight cases per 100 000, or in other words it has gone up. Of these eight cases:

  • There are five screen detected cases

  • There are three clinically diagnosed cases

◆ Death rate is two per 100 000, so is exactly the same

◆ Case survival in screen-detected cases is five out of five or 100 per cent, which sounds very impressive

◆ Case survival overall is six out of eight or 75 per cent, so has appeared to increase

◆ All the deaths occurred in cases that were undetected by screening.

If the case survival is taken out of context of the fact that your case definition has completely changed, then people are easily misled into believing that screening has truly been shown to improve survival—'All the cases picked up on screening survive, compared with only 33 per cent of non-screen-detected, and overall the survival in the population improves from 60 to 75 per cent!' This is exactly what is happening at present with prostate cancer. Widespread use of the prostate-specific antigen (PSA) test for screening is leading to a rise in incidence and in case survival, but this is because cases of inconsequential disease are being picked up and included in the statistics. Good outcome in screen-detected cases is being inappropriately interpreted as 'evidence' that screening does more good than harm.

Figure 4.1 also illustrates that the bias relates partly to the speed with which *clinical* cases progress, and partly to the overdiagnosis of *inconsequential* cases. It can be helpful to think of these as two separate biases—length time bias and overdiagnosis bias—but in practice they are hard to measure separately.

One way of visualizing pure length time bias is by imagining a disease where no inconsequential cases exist. The poor prognosis clinical cases tend to have a short symptomless phase. The window of opportunity for finding these cases on screening is very small. You have a better chance of picking up good prognosis clinical cases because they have slower progression and a longer symptomless phase. So your screen-detected cases are a particular subset of the clinical cases, with better prognosis, compared with all clinical cases diagnosed in the absence of screening. So that is the pure length time bias for clinical cases. Then, in addition to this, many screening tests pick up inconsequential disease, with the result that overdiagnosis bias adds to the length time effect.

It is important to use terms that are free of any built-in and possibly invalid assumptions concerning the past or future course of disease. Symptomless is not the same as pre-symptomatic, since pre-symptomatic implies that symptoms will definitely occur in the future. Symptomless is a preferable term because it means what it says—symptoms have not happened yet—but it leaves an open question as to whether they will. Similarly, the term 'early' is often used to describe screen-detected conditions, particularly cancers. What we really mean is that the cancer is localized and is not invading other tissues. How long it has been present, and what it will do in the future, is unknown. It may have been there for years and be at as late a stage as it will ever reach. So if we want to mean what we say we should call it localized not early. The word cancer itself is even problematic, as it is now abundantly clear that if any one of us had enough tissue samples taken and scrutinized carefully enough, we will somewhere have a bunch of cells that look like cancer cells. For a very clear explanation of how we know this, it is worth looking at Gilbert Welch's book *Should I be screened for cancer?* (Welch 2004).

Lead time effect

There is another bias that it is important to be aware of, and which was described in the 1960s when the need for RCTs of screening was first being articulated. It relates to the fact that survival time for people with screen-detected disease appears longer simply because you start the clock sooner. So if you imagine a person who has heart disease that will kill them when they are 55 years old exactly, and who is diagnosed clinically with heart disease when they are 54 years old exactly, then their survival time with heart disease is 1 year. Supposing instead that someone had screened them and found symptomless heart disease when they were 53 years old, but still they die at 55. The time they survive with heart disease is now 2 years just because you have added the 'lead in' time onto their recorded survival.

In practice, the effects of lead time and length time bias are difficult or impossible to measure separately, but the important message is that survival statistics must be treated with extreme caution. It is common to read in news stories that more men with prostate cancer are surviving, and surviving longer, than ever before, and that this is as a result of screening. However, all that is happening is that the survival time is being counted from the time of screen detection following PSA testing, and in addition many inconsequential cases are being added to the group classified as having cancer. If you look at Fig. 4.1 you can see how the survival time automatically increases because of screening, even if no-one benefits from screening.

For participants in screening, the effect is that they spend a greater part of their lives with knowledge of a disease, or pathological change, or risk marker, irrespective of whether they gain any real advantage in terms of longer life or less morbidity.

Three main methods for evaluating screening

Data affected by these three biases is not evidence. To find out whether screening really reduces risk of serious outcomes, you have to compare like with like in a well conducted RCT. This is the only source of reliable evidence about the consequences of screening. Carefully conducted time trend analyses can be valuable for looking at changes in death and incidence rates in a population once screening is happening but, without a truly comparable unscreened population for comparison, you are always left with uncertainty as to what the trends would have been had the screening not been introduced. Case–control studies can also be useful, particularly for comparing different policies and protocols, but they cannot reliably measure the difference between screening and no screening.

Randomized controlled trials (RCTs).

The basic method is:

- A population representative of those eligible for the screening is recruited then randomly assigned to different groups.

- One or more group is offered the intervention, i.e. the opportunity to participate in a screening programme. Different variations of screening protocol can be incorporated in the study design.

- The control group receives usual care.

- The same inclusion and exclusion criteria must be applied to all groups including the controls. The same rigour of follow-up and of establishing end-points, i.e. disease progression, death from the disease, etc., must be applied to all groups including the controls.

- All relevant outcomes are measured in both groups and compared.

- Meticulous care is needed in order to minimize the potential for bias. This applies to methods of recruitment, exclusions, randomization, achievement of complete follow-up, blinded ascertainment of diagnosis and blinded ascertainment of cause of death.

- The resources needed for screening are measured, in the research setting. This will tell you part of the costs, but provision of screening in a research trial does not include all the elements that have to be in place once a fully quality-assured and accessible programme is provided to the entire eligible population.

Important points about RCTs are:

- A major RCT yields data that are essential for policy and for the planning and implementation of a quality-assured programme.

- A major RCT is far less costly than unplanned growth of poor quality screening.

- The existence of a major RCT can discourage the haphazard growth of unplanned, non-evidence-based, poor quality delivery, with the harm that this entails.

- Tests and interventions can change during the life of an RCT. The study design needs to be capable of adopting important changes in screening methods should these become available.

- Economic analysis must avoid the fallacy of assuming that everyone saved by screening then dies of something that needs no care at all. Very often economists offset the cost of screening against the saving of treatment costs, without recognizing that treatment costs actually rise because of overdiagnosis, and that those who are helped by screening will need other types of care in the future. These errors lead to expectations that screening can be implemented with no resources.

- The widespread belief in the power of screening can make it difficult for potential participants to accept randomization, although this is changing.

- If there is widespread private provision of screening, particularly with direct-to-consumer advertising, there can be contamination of the control group. This makes it harder to detect any impact of screening reliably.

To illustrate with an example of a well designed RCT of screening, we can look at a trial of ovarian cancer screening that began recruitment in 2000.

Case 4.3 Case study—the UK Collaborative Trial of Ovarian Cancer Screening (UKCTOCS)

The benefit, harm and resources needed for ovarian cancer screening are unknown (Bell *et al.* 1998).

A large multicentre RCT of ovarian screening is therefore being conducted to establish what the consequences of ovarian screening actually are. It is funded jointly by four organizations. More information is on the trial's website (UK Collaborative Trial of Ovarian Cancer Screening website)

The objectives of the study as quoted on the website are:

- To establish the impact of ovarian screening on ovarian cancer mortality.
- To determine the physical morbidity of ovarian cancer screening.
- To determine the implications of screening on resources.
- To assess the feasibility of population screening as reflected by uptake of invitations and compliance with annual screening.
- To compare the performance of two screening strategies.
- To establish a serum bank for future assessment of novel tumour markers.

The study population is:

- 200 000 post-menopausal women age 50–74 recruited over the course of 3 years.

The source of recruitment is:

- Women are invited to participate from the age/sex registers of the local national health service administrative authorities, geographically related to the 13 regional collaborating centres.

The design is:

Women who agree to participate and who meet the inclusion criteria are then randomized to three groups.

- Two of the groups are offered annual screening. One group, 50 000 women, is offered screening using transvaginal ultrasound, the other group, 50 000 women, is offered screening

Case 4.3 Case study—the UK Collaborative Trial of Ovarian Cancer Screening (UKCTOCS) *(cont.)*

using a blood test to measure a tumour marker known as CA125, in addition to transvaginal ultrasound.

- The case definition for a screen-detected case is histologically confirmed ovarian cancer, although inevitably the study is uncovering localized non-invasive cancers and borderline conditions.

- In the ultrasound group, if a primary scan is positive, this is followed by a repeat scan 6 weeks later. If this second scan is also positive, then the woman goes on to the diagnostic stage, which involves laparoscopic surgery to remove her ovaries and fallopian tubes.

- In the CA125 group, sequential measurements are made. An algorithm based on data from women who developed clinical cancer is used to determine whether to proceed to the diagnostic stage of laparoscopic surgery to remove ovaries and fallopian tubes.

- The third group, 100 000 women, is not offered screening and receives usual care.

- Women with screen-detected cancer are referred to the specialist multidisciplinary gynaecological cancer team for treatment. These same teams will be treating any women from the control arm with clinically diagnosed cancer.

- All women in all three groups of the trial are followed-up in the same way through postal questionnaires and through the NHS Cancer Registry.

- A 1000 random sample of women in the study is included in the psychosocial arm of the study, designed to look at emotional, social and sexual effects of screening.

An important result will be the death rate from ovarian cancer in the offered screening group, compared with the death rate from ovarian cancer in the control group. Measures of the intervention rates and morbidity in the different groups will also be crucial, as there is a need to determine the overall balance of benefit and harm, and to document the overdiagnosis arising from screening.

Case 4.3 Case study—the UK Collaborative Trial of Ovarian Cancer Screening (UKCTOCS) *(cont.)*

Key challenges are ensuring there are minimal losses to follow-up, and independent assessors blinded as to which group women belonged to assigning the cause of death. Also, the psychosocial evaluation needs to look beyond the question of whether women feel grateful for the screening. Once you have been told you may have cancer, then your automatic reaction on learning you have had your ovaries removed unnecessarily is actually huge relief. Even where harm is definite and benefit non-existent there is ample evidence that people justify the unnecessary intervention by assuming that consequences for them would have been even worse without screening.

The need for proper RCT design and analysis may all seem rather obvious to many readers, particularly those of you with a background in scientific method, critical appraisal and epidemiology. However, it is worth emphasizing just how lacking this type of rigour has been in the world of screening. As an example, here is a case study concerning data that were published in a peer-reviewed journal claiming to be a report of an RCT, but which was not.

Case 4.4 Case study—flawed analysis from a randomized trial, the Labrie study from Quebec

In 1988 in Quebec City, Canada, the electoral rolls were used to obtain details of men aged 45–80 for recruitment to a prostate cancer detection study. After exclusion of 536 men who had already been screened or who had already been diagnosed with prostate cancer, there were 46 193 men deemed eligible for the study.

◆ The eligible participants assigned to the intervention group comprised 30 956 men who were sent letters inviting them for annual screening.

◆ The eligible participants assigned to the control group comprised 15 237 men who were not invited.

Case 4.4 Case study—flawed analysis from a randomized trial, the Labrie study from Quebec *(cont.)*

- Assignment to the two groups was random.

- Cause-specific death data were obtained from the Death Registry of the Health Department of the Province of Quebec for the 8 year period 1989–1996.

A paper describing first results from the study was published in 1999 in the journal *The Prostate* (Labrie *et al.* 1999). Careful reading of this paper shows that:

- In the group offered screening, 7155 men (23.1 per cent) attended at least once for screening.

- In the control group, 982 men (6.4 per cent) attended for screening even though they were not invited. This phenomenon is known as 'contamination' of the control group and is unavoidable where screening is widely promoted and accessible.

- The death rates from prostate cancer in the intervention group and the control groups were similar, with 97 prostate cancer deaths among the 30 965 invited men, and 45 prostate cancer deaths among the 15 237 uninvited men (crude rates are 3.13 and 2.95 per 10 000, respectively).

- The authors present figures relating to person years at risk, and again there is no difference between the invited and the uninvited groups.

- The results of the study therefore show no measurable impact on prostate cancer mortality from a 23.1 per cent uptake of screening in 30 956 invited men compared with 6.4 per cent screening in 15 237 uninvited men.

Yet the paper actually concludes that the results of the RCT demonstrate that screening brings a 'dramatic' decrease in prostate cancer deaths. The authors decided to ignore their randomization, and their exclusion criteria. Their analysis compares the death rate in men in either arm of the trial who declined screening, with those in either arm of the trial who accepted screening. Not surprisingly, given what we know about the healthy screenee effect, the prostate

Case 4.4 Case study—flawed analysis from a randomized trial, the Labrie study from Quebec *(cont.)*

cancer death rate in the men who self-selected to be screened was substantially lower than in those who self-selected to decline screening. The paper claims to include an 'intent-to-treat' analysis, which is the technical term for analysing the groups as randomized irrespective of compliance with the intervention. The way the results are described and presented is very confusing, but the authors' idea of an intent-to-treat analysis does not seem to match any standard method.

Letters to the journal pointed out in no uncertain terms that the analysis was entirely invalid and that the study provided no evidence of an impact on prostate cancer deaths (Alexander and Prescott 1999; Boer and Schroder 1999), though the replies from the study authors continued to reiterate a maze of confusing and irrelevant statistics.

Astonishingly, in 2004, *The Prostate* published a second paper from the same study, again with flawed analysis, again showing no impact on mortality but claiming a major effect (Labrie *et al.* 2004). Again there was criticism from around the world (Barratt and Coates 2004; Elwood 2004; Pinsky 2004). *The Prostate* submits all papers for peer review, but the arrangements for ensuring scientific robustness are clearly inadequate. When we inquired as to how statistics and methods are assessed before publication, we were simply referred to their website, which gives only the sketchiest information.

Before we leave the topic of RCTs, it is important to acknowledge that there are circumstances where it can be very difficult to do such a trial, and some circumstances where it is impossible.

♦ For very rare diseases, the size of controlled trial needed may be prohibitive, but alternative research designs can nevertheless be implemented. For very rare disorders in newborn babies for example, it can be feasible to enroll infants in studies even without a formal randomized trial. A recent paper in the American journal *Pediatrics* (Botkin *et al.* 2006) stresses the need for this approach, and makes justifiably strong criticism of recent recommendations from the American College of Medical Genetics concerning expansion of newborn screening—based, like the 1957 Commission on Chronic Illness recommendations (see Chapter 1, p. 11), on opinion and no evidence (US Department of Health and Human Services 2005).

◆ Where professionals are convinced of the benefit from screening, it may also be difficult to do the necessary research, as Archie Cochrane found in relation to cervical screening in the 1960s (see Chapter 1, p. 20) although in retrospect Cochrane was right and proper trials would have avoided huge waste of resources and considerable harm to women.

Time trend studies

The basic method in a time trend study is:

◆ Observation, and analysis, once screening is in place, of trends over time in measures of disease frequency, such as incidence and deaths.

◆ Data should be for a long time period starting well before screening began so that the background trend is clear.

◆ It is important to examine separately the trends in different age groups and, for some diseases, different birth cohorts.

◆ Objective measures of screening coverage and screening quality, for different age groups and cohorts, should be assessed and analysed alongside the death and incidence trend data.

◆ Sources of bias such as variation in ascertainment, or changes in diagnostic practice, should be properly considered.

◆ Other influences on rates such as advances in treatment or reduction in co-morbidity should be properly considered.

◆ If numbers are small then statistical tests should be used to distinguish ordinary variation from significant change.

◆ Wherever possible there should be comparison with equivalent trend data for a comparable country or region that does not have a screening programme. In effect this takes the study design beyond that of just a time trend analysis, as it incorporates a geographical comparison.

Important points about time trend studies are:

+ If screening begins without RCT evidence, then time trend analysis may be the only way of examining any impact of screening on disease and deaths.

+ When screening is implemented because of RCT evidence, then time trend analysis is a means of estimating whether the predicted impact appears to be being realized.

+ It can never be known for certain what would have happened to trends had screening not been introduced

+ Measures of disease frequency are subject to a range of inaccuracies and sources of bias.

+ Measures of disease frequency are themselves influenced by screening, because greater awareness and publicity can lead to an increased likelihood of disease registration or of recording on death certification, and because latent disease is uncovered and labelled as disease.

+ Published time trend studies, even in peer-reviewed journals, are sometimes very poor quality. For example, they may be based on small numbers, short time periods and with no objective measures of what constitutes a high quality screening programme. An example is the much-quoted *Lancet* paper that showed the 'Iceland effect'—an apparent instant 80 per cent drop in deaths from cervical cancer during 1965–1981 due to 'well organized' screening in Iceland (Laara *et al.* 1987). This was based on tiny numbers and a short time period; in effect, the *Lancet* paper simply reported one spike amidst ordinary small number variation. It also overlooked the fact that by 1981 only 50 per cent of the eligible population in Iceland had been screened (Sigurdsson *et al.* 1989) so even if screening were 100 per cent effective this could only have cut deaths by 50 per cent. Mortality in Iceland has indeed fallen, but a comprehensive overview of cervical cancer trends in European countries shows a complex picture (Levi *et al.* 2000). The strongest time trend evidence for cervical screening comes from analysis by birth cohorts, as published for England and Wales by Peter Sasieni and colleagues (Sasieni *et al.* 1995; Sasieni and Adams 1999; Quinn *et al.* 1999), and from rising mortality in countries such as Ireland where quality-assured screening has only recently been established (Levi *et al.* 2000).

Case 4.5 Case study—prostate cancer mortality time trends in different countries

Falling mortality rates from prostate cancer were being quoted as 'evidence' that the widespread adoption of PSA testing in the USA was improving men's health. Other countries, without widespread use of PSA were seeing similar trends. Oliver and colleagues therefore set out to analyse and report, in a consistent way, mortality data from as many different countries as possible (Oliver *et al.* 2001). This paper avoided the mistakes made in many of the cervical cancer time trend reports of the 1970s:

- Data for prostate cancer deaths from 1979 to 1997 were extracted from the World Health Organization database
- The criteria for selecting countries to include in the analysis were stated
- The method of analysing mortality trends was described
- The possible influences of artefact, changes in underlying incidence, changes in competing mortality and changes in survival due to treatment service improvements were discussed
- Referenced comment on the intensity of PSA screening in the nations studied was included in the Discussion
- Conclusions were suitably cautious, and the limitations of time trend analysis were stated.

Case–control studies

The basic method for a case–control study of screening is:

- A clear case definition is agreed. This must be a case definition that comprises subjects with the outcome that screening is aiming to prevent. So for example the case definition must include serious and fatal cases. A time period, a geographical area and a source population that is eligible to be screened are chosen. Every case of the disease arising during that time in the source population resident in that place, including fatalities, is identified. Complete ascertainment is important. Assignment of cause of death should be based on examination of case records not just death certification.

◆ For each case, one or more controls drawn from the same source population is identified. Controls must be comparable with the cases, so controls are usually matched for age, sex, place of residence and other known risk factors if possible.

◆ A definition is drawn up of what constitutes participation in screening, and how to separate tests done as screening from tests done because the disease was already symptomatic. Records of past participation in screening are obtained and validated for all cases and controls. It is not reliable just to ask the study participants if they can remember being screened.

◆ Participation in screening is compared between cases and controls. If participation is higher in controls than in cases, this gives a suggestion that screening may reduce risk. It does not give certain evidence because it may be that the result is due to confounding. In other words, factors that make you less likely to develop serious disease, for example education, good existing health and high income, also make you more likely to have screening. The aim of matching is to reduce confounding, but it cannot eliminate it. (You have probably spotted that this is the healthy screenee effect at work again.)

Important points about case control studies are:

◆ The methodology is a tricky subject, see for example the review of Cronin *et al.* (1998) of theory and practice.

◆ If screening is already in place and there is variation in practice, then case–control studies may be the only way of trying to compare factors such as screening frequency.

◆ Published case–control studies, even in peer-reviewed journals, are sometimes very poor quality. For example, they may be based on small numbers, poor case definition, poor definition of source population and time period, they may rely only on participant's memory of whether they had screening, and there may be no attempt to ensure that all cases including fatalities are captured. Results must always be treated with extreme caution, and if any of the above factors apply they should be regarded as useless.

♦ For some screening, we have the benefit of evidence from case–control studies and RCTs, and time trend analysis. This demonstrates that case–control studies generally tend to overestimate the effect of screening and should be treated with caution (Moss 1991).

Case 4.6 Case study—breast self-examination

This case study is about breast self-examination. The screening test, or sieve, is self-examination, and the diagnostic phase, the sort, is investigation at a dedicated breast screening unit for any problems found. The aim is to reduce risk of death from breast cancer. A case–control study was carried out in Nottingham, UK to examine the effect of education about breast self-examination (Locker 1989).

♦ The Nottingham breast self-examination education programme began from 1979 and invited women to attend the screening unit for education about breast self-examination. Women who attended the education could subsequently contact the screening units directly should they find any problems with their breasts.

♦ The cases in the case–control study were women who died of breast cancer between 1979 and 1987, and who had been included in the Nottingham breast self-examination project. It is important in case–control design to ensure that the cases are representative of those who suffer the bad outcome that the intervention aims to prevent, so the Nottingham study fulfilled this.

♦ Controls were women in the same age group and the same family doctor practice who had been included in the breast self-examination education project and who had not died of breast cancer.

Case 4.6 Case study—breast self-examination *(cont.)*

- Exposure to the intervention was then ascertained by checking the attendance registers to see which women had attended for breast self-examination education. This is also important, as it validates the exposure, and does not rely on subjects' or relatives' memory as to whether the participation happened.

The study findings were:

- Among 201 cases (women who died of breast cancer) there were 80 (39.8 per cent) who had attended the education about breast self-examination. Among 603 controls there were 292 (48.4 per cent) who had attended the education about breast self-examination. So there was an association between not attending for education, and dying of breast cancer.

- This works out as a relative risk of 0.7, with a 95 per cent confidence interval of 0.5–0.97. In other words, in the 804 women in this study, the risk of dying of breast cancer in the women who attended education was only 70 per cent of the risk of dying of breast cancer in the women who did not attend. The fact that the upper end of the confidence interval is below 1 indicates that this difference has only a 1 in 20 likelihood of being a purely chance finding. When the results for post-menopausal women were analysed separately, it was found that the relative risk in post-menopausal women who had attended education was even lower at 0.66.

- The authors concluded that the case–control study demonstrated the value of attendance for education in breast self-examination particularly in post-menopausal women.

The weakness with this conclusion is that it assumes that the relationship between attending for education and risk of dying of breast cancer is entirely causal. It ignores the possibility that there could be confounding factors. Confounders are things that are linked both to lower risk of breast cancer death and to likelihood of attending. The matching of the controls, by selecting each control from the same family doctor practice as the case, aims to reduce the effect of confounders, but it cannot guarantee comparable groups in the way that randomization can.

Case 4.6 Case study—breast self-examination *(cont.)*

Even at the time of publication, the authors might have been less inclined to draw their conclusion if they had taken account of the fact that overall, the death rates from breast cancer in the two locations that were running breast self-examination education (Nottingham and Huddersfield) were higher than in comparison districts where breast self-examination was not being taught (UKTEDBC 1988). If the claimed 30 per cent cut in deaths amongst the 49 cent of the study population who attended had been genuine, then the death rate should have been lower, but it was not. The authors ignored this fact and instead they supported their conclusion with the fact that a greater proportion of the breast cancers in the women who attended for education were small and low grade, compared with a historical control group. However, as you will know from the earlier part of the chapter, this is to be expected because self-examination is a form of screening, and screen-detected cases are likely to differ from clinically presenting cases because of length time bias and overdiagnosis bias.

There has now been an RCT trial comparing breast cancer death rates in women offered intensive education in breast self-examination, and control women not offered this. The mortality in the two groups was the same (Thomas *et al.* 2000). This study was performed in China, and one has to be somewhat cautious about assuming that interventions, diagnostic criteria and study design are directly comparable across continents. Nevertheless, this does add strong weight to the likelihood that the observed positive result in the Nottingham self-examination case–control study was a result of confounding factors. So what this shows us is that even with a screening intervention that when tested by RCT gives no benefit, there is a good chance that a case–control study could 'find' an apparent effect.

Two additional sources of information

Once you have evidence from RCTs that screening will do more good than harm, then pilot projects and modelling studies can yield valuable information.

Pilot/demonstration projects

In a pilot project you try out screening on a limited scale and evaluate what happens.

This approach can be used to:

- Solve practical problems and learn lessons concerning the implementation of screening (see also Chapter 5).

- Work out the resources needed to deliver a programme in an ordinary service setting.

- Test out arrangements such as training for staff, information and support for participants, how to deal with uncertain categories of disease, systems for information management and technology, and quality management (see also Chapter 6).

Case 4.7 Case study—piloting liquid-based cytology in English cervical screening laboratories

- Three pilot laboratories in England were used to test out the effects, in the English cervical screening programme, of using liquid-based cytology in place of conventional cytology for cervical screening (National Institute for Clinical Excellence 2003).

- With liquid-based cytology, the cell sample is placed, by the sample taker, into a vial of liquid and a cleaned cell sample is prepared in the laboratory for visual inspection. With conventional cytology, the sample is spread on a glass slide by the sample taker and covered with a chemical fixative before sending it to the laboratory for staining and visual inspection.

Case 4.7 Case study—piloting liquid-based cytology in English cervical screening laboratories *(cont.)*

- The pilot aim was not to evaluate liquid-based cytology in relation to outcome measures such as cancers prevented, it simply aimed to determine whether in NHS laboratories it could meet equivalent quality standards to conventional cytology and reduce the number of tests that were judged inadequate and in need of repeating.

- The pilot enabled information to be collected about test performance, technical performance of the equipment, training requirements and resources needed. The pilot also meant that laboratory staff, sample takers and screening participants could be asked what difference the change in test method made for them.

- The result was a national decision to roll-out liquid-based cytology to all laboratories over the course of 5 years. One reason for this decision was that the percentage of tests judged adequate rose to over 99 per cent compared with around 88 per cent using conventional cytology. This represents a very substantial number of women who do not have to have the test repeated. Inadequate rates vary substantially from nation to nation, for many reasons, so a pilot specific to UK NHS practice was therefore valuable. The second main benefit was that throughput increased.

- The rate-limiting step in rolling out the technology is the capacity of regional training centres to train all the sample readers in using the new technique. The pilot enabled robust plans to be made.

- One limitation in the evaluation of the pilot was that the economic analysis was very unsatisfactory and did not give clear and realistic information about the actual running costs. Instead, a complex modelling technique offset the manufacturers price per test against the saving of a few minutes of sample takers' time, leading to the mistaken conclusion that no extra revenue funding was needed for implementation.

Modelling studies

These are studies that take evidence gathered from different sources and test out different scenarios relating for example to uptake, definition of eligible group, frequency of testing or threshold for intervention. They attempt to make an overall prediction of outcomes and costs for a theoretical screened population given varying parameters.

One example is a study examining the potential benefit of adding automated techniques for cervical cytology testing into the existing cervical screening programme for the UK (Willis *et al.* 2005). The literature provides some data about test performance for these new technologies, and about cost. To translate this into predicted benefits and harms for women, you have to do a modelling study but, even with the vast experience we have of delivering cervical screening, many assumptions have to be made to produce a model.

Measures of test performance

Measurement of test performance is a complex subject in its own right. In this section, we give the basics. If you need more depth on these matters, we recommend Raj Bhopal's book *Concepts of epidemiology and integrated introduction to the ideas, theories, principles and methods of epidemiology* (Bhopal 2002).

There are many questions to be grappled with, including:

◆ Does the test give a valid, reliable and accurate measure of the thing you want to measure?

◆ Is there variation between different observers, and between different measurements done by the same observer, and what can be done to keep this variation to a minimum?

◆ Given that most measured variables are continuously distributed, what cut-off should be used to divide measurements into two categories, positive and negative? By 'continuously distributed' we mean that the categories merge into each other (is this banana ripe or not ripe), as opposed to a categorical difference (is this a banana or a pineapple).

Assessing test performance is important in screening programmes, as is the establishment of quality management systems (see Chapter 6) to ensure optimum test performance. However, measures of test performance do not in themselves tell you anything about what benefit and harm will result from the screening programme.

The basic measures of test performance are sensitivity, specificity, positive predictive value, negative predictive value and receiver operating characteristic curves (ROC curves).

Test sensitivity and specificity

Sensitivity is the ability of a test to detect the condition that the test is measuring for when, in fact, it is present.

For example, the sensitivity of a cervical cytology test is its ability to detect cervical intraepithelial neoplasia (CIN) as defined by histological examination of a tissue sample.

Specificity is the ability of a test to detect that the condition being measured for by the test is not present when it is, in fact, not present.

True positives have the condition being measured for by the test, and the test result is positive. True negatives do not have the condition being measured for by the test, and the test result is negative.

The calculation of test sensitivity and specificity is shown in Table 4.1.

$$\text{Sensitivity} = A/A + C.$$

$$\text{Specificity} = D/B + D.$$

Table 4.1 Calculation of test sensitivity and specificity

		Condition being tested for		
		Present	*Absent*	*Totals*
Test result	*Positive*	A: true positives	B: false positives	A + B
	Negative	C: false negatives	D: true negatives	C + D
	Totals	A + C	B + D	A + B + C + D

Positive and negative predictive values

The positive predictive value of a test is the probability that an individual has the condition being tested for, given that the result is positive.

The negative predictive value of a test is the probability that an individual does not have the condition being tested for, given that the result is negative.

Using the two by two table, the calculations are:

Positive predictive value = A/A + B

Negative predictive value = D/C + D

Yet again, it is crucial to be absolutely clear what you mean by the *condition* being tested for, or in other words what is your case definition for this test. If, for example, you are measuring blood pressure, then your case definition for quantifying test performance might be blood pressure raised above a certain level, and verified by a certain number of repeat tests. The blood pressure test is measuring a risk marker, and its performance is expressed as the accuracy with which it measures that risk marker. The risk marker is not the same as the condition that the screening programme is aiming to ameliorate, which in the example of blood pressure would be stroke.

Positive and negative predictive values are profoundly influenced by the prevalence of the condition in the group being tested or, in other words, by the risk or 'pre-test probability' in the person being tested. The same test will produce vastly better predictive values when applied in a high prevalence group than when it is applied in a low prevalence group. This is the main reason why hospital doctors believe that family doctors miss 'easy' diagnoses, and why family doctors believe that hospital doctors overinvestigate.

The best way of understanding this is to work out an example for yourself, and question three in the test yourself section at the end of this chapter gives you an example.

What is happening here is the same phenomenon that underlies the use of pre-test probability, post-test probability and odds ratios for expressing the usefulness of diagnostic tests.

Receiver operator characteristic curves

An ROC curve is a way of illustrating, on one graph, and for one test, the sensitivity and specificity achieved at any cut-off level and the trade-off between them. It helps you assess your test, and helps you choose the cut-off. It is probably fair to say that only the very statistically minded find them easy to understand, and even the name is confusing, as sometimes they are called 'receiver operator characteristic' and sometimes 'receiver operating characteristic' and sometimes just 'receiver operator curve'. According to Wikipedia, the name dates back to the aftermath of the Japanese attack on the US Navy in Pearl Harbour in 1941. Investigators wanted to see how it was that the personnel operating the radar receivers (the receiver operators) had been unable to distinguish the Japanese planes from all the other signals they were getting. They used ROC curves as a method of summarizing the performance of an operator in discriminating between different signals, so that they could study the effects of different conditions, signals, and so on.

Traditionally the y-axis shows the sensitivity, or, put in other words, 1 – the false-negative rate. These are expressed not in the usual format of percentages, but as proportions of 1. So 80 per cent sensitivity will appear as 0.8, and this is the same as saying that the fals-negative rate is 20 per cent or 0.2, hence 1 – false negatives is 0.8.

The x-axis shows 1 – the specificity, or in other words the false-positive rate. So 80 per cent specificity will appear as 1 – 0.8, so 0.2. This is the same as saying that the false-positive rate is 20 per cent or 0.2.

The curve for a test with high sensitivity and specificity will hug the left hand and top sides of the square, and will have an area under the curve approaching 1. The curve for a useless test, equivalent to tossing a coin to see if someone is positive or negative, goes straight from the bottom left hand corner to the top right hand corner, and the area under the curve is 0.5.

Figure 4.2 shows an example of a ROC curve.

ROC curves are a useful way of displaying data about test performance, but they do not tell you anything about whether the screening programme will do more good than harm.

Summarizing all information on outcomes

Screening programmes have a range of consequences for the population screened. Once you have evidence about all the important outcomes, you need to present this information in a way that can be readily understood.

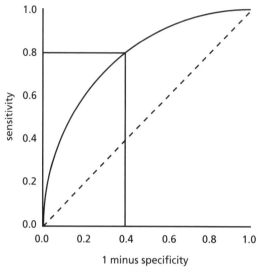

Fig. 4.2 A 'receiver operator characteristic' curve. The solid curve is for a test that achieves 80 per cent sensitivity with 60 per cent specificity. The dashed curve is for a test that is no better than tossing a coin.

- It is not adequate to describe only the harmful effects or only the beneficial effects.

- Nor is it adequate to present information only as relative risks, or statistical probabilities, such that only a postgraduate statistician with time to spare would be able to work out real numbers in a screened population.

The numbers in the flow diagram

Increasingly the outcomes of screening are being presented in a way that matches the flow diagram used in Chapters 2 and 3 (see p. 78). This is like using a care pathway for an individual patient, but in this case the patient is a whole population. So the diagram is in effect a population care pathway for screening. The information is helpful for planning the service, and it is essential for preparing information for potential participants. Here is an example relating to bowel cancer screening.

Case 4.8 Case study—the numbers in the flow diagram for bowel cancer screening (See Fig. 4.3, p. 122)

In 1998, as part of the planning stages for bowel cancer screening in the UK, the Health Economics Research Unit at Oxford University was commissioned to prepare information about the numbers of people that would be going through the different stages of the screening system, and the outcomes (National Screening Committee 1998). They used data summarized from published bowel screening studies (Hardcastle *et al.* 1996; Kronberg *et al.* 1996; Winawer *et al.* 1997) and computed the outcomes for 100 000 men and women aged 50–69. This is not a simple exercise, and their report covers 16 pages. The results enable us to fill in most of the elements in the screening flow diagram. This is shown in Fig. 4.3 (see p. 122).

- The screening test, or sieve, is called the 'faecal occult blood test' or FOBT, which is sent to participants for them to do at home and mail back the completed test.

- The diagnostic investigation, or sort, involves examination of the inside of the bowel using a fibreoptic tube. This is called colonoscopy. The patient takes laxatives the day before to prepare the bowel, and the procedure is done as a day case and does not need general anaesthetic.

- Any abnormalities found can be biopsied to remove a piece of tissue for histological examination in a pathology laboratory.

- If benign growths, known as polyps, are found, then these are removed during the colonoscopy investigation, and the polyps are examined histologically in a pathology laboratory.

- The complications of colonoscopy are that rarely (8 per 100 000 colonoscopies in a high quality service) a patient bleeds from the bowel, or a hole is caused in the bowel. Both these complications can result in the patient staying in hospital, and possibly having an operation to stop the bleeding or to repair the perforation. Most of the complications are in patients who have polyps removed during their colonoscopy.

Case 4.8 Case study—the numbers in the flow diagram for bowel cancer screening (cont.)

♦ If an invading cancer is found, then the appropriate intervention is for the patient to have planned surgery to remove the tumour, together with treatment using cancer drugs. Complications from cancer treatment are not included in Fig. 4.3.

As with all screening programmes, the numbers in the flow diagram highlight some important consequences and uncertainties:

♦ Once symptomless people have colonoscopy it turns out that many people have intestinal polyps. These are smooth growths protruding from the interior of the intestinal wall. They are also called adenomas. Histological examination of polyp tissue shows that some contain cells that look like cancer cells, and some show microscopic evidence that the cancer cells are behaving like cancer cells and invading into surrounding tissue. As with other organs (see pp. 26, 72, 96, 185), there is a problem in knowing exactly what we mean by cancer cells, as the truth seems to be that all of us have cells somewhere that look like cancer but are not behaving like cancer, and the harder you look the more you find. The classification of cells as suspicious or not is subjective, and different pathologists have different thresholds. Some adenomatous polyps will progress to become clinically invasive cancer, but what proportion of polyps progress during the person's lifetime, and which ones, is unknown.

♦ Literature from Japan and the USA shows that once routine colonoscopy is used as a screening method, the number of people with polyps detected grows. Published rates vary according to the classification used, whether flat adenomas are included, the investigation used and the study population. The estimate of one to two hundred cases treated for inconsequential disease was based on USA data (Winawer *et al.* 1997). The estimate of around 30 cases categorized as suspicious and followed-up was based on estimates from pathologists involved in the screening trials, suggesting that 5 per cent of polyps are found to have severe dysplasia.

Case 4.8 Case study—the numbers in the flow diagram for bowel cancer screening *(cont.)*

- It is not easy to determine from the published data the exact split, in the intervention group, between those who do well but would have done well without screening, and those who do badly despite screening. So the figure shows the 35 who as a result of screening have their life expectancy prolonged, and the 82 where screening makes no difference. Some of the 82 will do very well, and some will not.

- Sometimes it is argued that most of the hundreds of cases with polyps removed have cancer and cancer death prevented as a result. However, any colorectal cancer deaths prevented must show up as the mortality difference found in the trials between the offered screening and the control group, so they form part of the 35 people benefited. Therefore, most of the patients with polyps removed have inconsequential disease.

- Results of well conducted RCTs show the benefit in a group offered screening, compared with a group not offered screening. Adjusting this to give a benefit in 100 000 who actually participate inevitably requires some approximation.

The work shown in Fig. 4.3 was done in 1998, before the UK bowel screening pilot sites were established. It was helpful not only for planning, but also for raising important questions about informed choice. At the planning workshops run by the National Screening Committee, some people argued that only the benefits should be explained to participants, whilst others argued that the potential risks must be made explicit (Raffle 2000).

The bowel cancer screening pilot sites in Scotland and England have now published their experience, and this has proved to be similar to the 1988 predictions. Data from the pilot sites (UK Colorectal Cancer Screening Pilot Group 2004) are shown below in order to enable comparison with Fig. 4.3:

In the UK bowel screening pilot sites, for each 100 000 who completed the FOBT:

- 1859 had a positive FOBT result
- 1515 accepted colonoscopy

Case 4.8 Case study—the numbers in the flow diagram for bowel cancer screening *(cont.)*

- 1362 completed colonoscopy, and 147 needed barium enema examination because of incomplete colonoscopy

- 169 had colorectal cancer diagnosed and treated with colectomy

- 34 had invasive polyps diagnosed, removed at colonoscopy and followed-up

- 511 had adenomatous polyps, not suspicious, diagnosed and removed at colonoscopy

- eight patients stayed overnight, or were readmitted to hospital because of pain or bleeding following colonoscopy, and one suffered perforation of the colon from polypectomy.

As mentioned on p. 63 (the polyp puzzle), clarity about pathological criteria for defining 'invasive' and 'suspicious' polyps, and about the real risk of progression during the patient's lifetime, is still unclear.

Information for participants

It is only relatively recently that researchers have started working with service users to develop ways of presenting full information in a format that can be used by people deciding whether to undergo screening. Previously it was felt that informed choice was not important because everyone should just be screened. This was mainly because the potential adverse effects of screening were barely recognized, and partly because comprehensive coverage had proved hard to achieve so information was used to encourage people to come. We return to this issue in Chapter 8 (see p. 249).

User-friendly leaflets, flow diagrams and decision aids are now beginning to be developed and tested. There is clear evidence (Gigerenzer 2002) that information is best understood if presented as simple frequencies, for example 'if 10 000 people like you are screened regularly for ten years, 40 will have surgery for a screen-detected condition and of those one will be saved from dying' (see also p. 221). Key principles for what constitutes a good quality decision aid are being established internationally (Elwyn *et al.* 2006). There is still

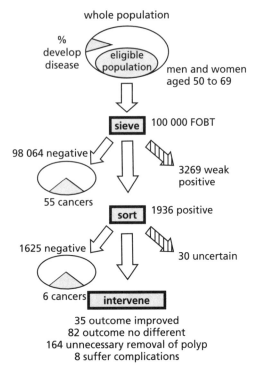

Fig. 4.3 The numbers in the flow diagram for bowel cancer screening (information used in 1998 for planning the UK bowel screening pilots).

a lot to be learned about the best ways of explaining screening. The lead time effect and the length time effect are concepts that have been little shared with the general public and with participants, but they need to be.

Summary points

Healthy people are more likely to get screened than less healthy people. This bias is known as the healthy screenee effect, and means that outcome in screened people looks good even if screening makes no difference.

Summary points *(cont.)*

Screening is more likely to pick up cases that stay symptomless for a long time and less likely to pick up rapidly progressive disease. This means that cases found by screening are a different group compared with cases that present clinically. They automatically have better prognosis, even if screening makes no difference, compared with disease that presents with symptoms. This bias is called length time bias.

Screening for risk markers or detectable pathological changes often uncovers inconsequential cases that would have no clinical impact in the person's lifetime. These cases are a different group compared with cases that present clinically. They have excellent prognosis, and screening leads to the person receiving diagnosis and treatment that they would not otherwise have. The incorporation of inconsequential cases makes outcome in a screen-detected group appear very good. This bias is called overdiagnosis bias.

Well conducted RCTs are the best source of reliable evidence about the difference made by screening.

Case–control studies of screening have many methodological pitfalls, and their results should be treated with extreme caution.

Time trend analysis of deaths can be valuable if used carefully. Time trends in incidence are less useful because definitions and ascertainment vary.

Pilot/demonstration studies can answer questions about implementation and the needs for resources.

Modelling studies can test out different scenarios for screening policy and protocol.

Economic analysis should be practical and realistic. It is a fallacy to offset screening costs with saved treatment costs since this assumes that all people helped by screening die of diseases that need zero care.

Test performance can be expressed as sensitivity, specificity, predictive values and receiver operating characteristic (ROC) curves. These are important but tell you nothing about the impact of a screening programme.

> **Summary points** *(cont.)*
>
> To describe all the consequences of screening properly, the evidence about benefits and harms should be summarized as simple frequencies. This can be done using a flow diagram for a screened population.
>
> Development of comprehensive information for potential participants is a relatively new venture, but is progressing.

Test yourself

Question one

You are peer reviewing a report submitted for publication in a scientific journal. It describes a controlled trial of lung cancer screening.

- The randomization was by geographical area, with the control group made up of all resident people in an area demographically comparable with the intervention group area.
- Everyone living in the intervention group area and registered with a family doctor was included in the intervention group and was written to and invited for screening.
- Those who responded to the researchers letter but who already had lung cancer were excluded from any further analysis.
- People living in the control area were the controls. They were not written to. In control subjects, all deaths from lung cancer during the study period were ascertained from death certificates by means of postcode of residence.
- The researchers ascertained cause of death in the study group by scrutiny of case notes.

What main concerns about bias would you raise in your comments to the editors?

Question two

An exercise electrocardiogram involves recording a person's heart trace (ECG) whilst they exercise on a treadmill. It is used in people with symptoms of heart disease, to learn more about the nature and severity of their problem. Abnormal findings are an indication that the blood supply to the heart muscle may be impaired. Technical criteria, relating to the degree of elevation of certain parts of the trace, determine the cut-off for defining an abnormal result.

Imagine you are considering using the exercise ECG as a screening test in symptomless people, in order to identify people who might have coronary heart disease (CHD), defined as significant impairment of the blood supply to the heart muscle, and who might benefit from early intervention. The exercise test has a sensitivity for detecting coronary heart disease of around 50 per cent and a specificity of around 90 per cent (Gibbons *et al.* 2002). Supposing the prevalence of CHD in symptomless people in their 50s is 5 per cent:

(a) Among 10 000 symptomless people in their 50s, who have not been tested, how many will have undiagnosed coronary heart disease?

(b) Now draw up a two by two table (see p. 114) and work out the numbers that fall into each of the boxes (true positives, false positives, etc.) if they all undergo the exercise ECG test.

(c) How many people have a positive exercise ECG result but do not have coronary heart disease?

(d) How many have a negative exercise ECG result but do have coronary heart disease?

(e) What is the positive predictive value (this is the probability that a person with a positive result actually has coronary heart disease—the formula is A divided by A + B. It can also be expressed as a percentage by multiplying by 100)

(f) What do you think are the reasons that exercise ECG is not recommended for screening symptomless people?

Question three

Imagine that you are applying the same exercise ECG test, with sensitivity of 50 per cent and specificity of 90 per cent for picking up CHD, but this time the underlying prevalence of CHD in the population you are testing is 1 per cent instead of 5 per cent.

(a) Draw up a two by two table and work out the numbers in each box, but this time for a prevalence of 1 per cent.

(b) Work out the positive predictive value using the formula A/A + B.

(c) Compare this with the positive predictive value for the example in question two.

(d) What effect has the prevalence had on the test performance, as expressed by the positive predictive value?

Question four

Each year in your local population 100 people are diagnosed with lung cancer, 80 of whom are dead within 1 year of diagnosis.

(a) what percentage of cases survive at 1 year, and what percentage of cases are dead at 1 year?

Screening for lung cancer is introduced. In the majority of screen-detected cases, the cancer-like changes are confined to the bronchial epithelium, these are classified as 'early' lung cancer and are seen as a sign that the screening is successfully picking up the cases before they spread. Ten years after the introduction of screening, the situation is as follows. Each year in your local population you now have 150 people diagnosed with lung cancer, 80 of whom are dead within 1 year of diagnosis.

(b) What percentage of cases survive at 1 year, and what percentage of cases are dead at 1 year?

(c) Has the number of people dying of lung cancer changed?

(d) What will have happened to the statistics on proportion diagnosed at an 'early' stage?

The many 'survivors' with localized cancer picked up on screening form a pressure group to campaign for the screening to be extended to other areas

(e) What would you recommend should happen?

Chapter 5

Implementing screening

The aim of the chapter

This chapter aims to give you an understanding of the essential tasks involved in setting up a good quality screening programme.

There is an old saying that all you have to do to create an effective service is:

- choose the right things to do, then

- do them right.

Choosing the right screening involves assessing the evidence (Chapter 4) and making policy (Chapter 8). Doing screening right means setting up a well ordered programme when screening is worthwhile (this chapter), ensuring that the service is always of high quality (Chapter 6), dealing effectively with problems (Chapter 7) and making sure that when harm is more likely than benefit then screening does not happen (Chapter 7).

Different healthcare systems have very different ways of planning, delivering, and funding their screening programmes (see also Chapter 2, p. 50). The UK currently has centralized policy making and decentralized provision. A diverse range of provider organizations deliver the screening services to the 57 million population, with a complex and changing pattern of accountabilities and funding mechanisms underpinning these arrangements. In every region and every district there is a director of public health, responsible for the health of his or her population. This provides a means of ensuring a population approach to local implementation and co-ordination of screening services, and to the monitoring and management of quality and performance. In this chapter, we try to focus on matters that are essential if screening is to achieve public health improvement—irrespective of where, and in what type of health system, it is being delivered.

For international readers, you will find that some of our organization descriptions and jargon need translating to apply them to your local setting, but we hope that the fundamental issues will be recognizable to all.

Drivers for unplanned screening

Before we look at how to start a programme, it is worth considering why it is that sometimes screening starts on its own and sometimes it waits for national implementation. Two major factors influencing this are the accessibility of the tests and the incentives within the health system.

Accessibility of tests

♦ Some screening tests can easily creep into practice because it is easy to start using them for symptomless people. Blood tests such as the prostate-specific antigen (PSA) test are an example.

♦ Other tests are less accessible, particularly if they need specialized equipment and trained operators. Examples are mammography breast X-rays, and screening for newborn babies using oto-acoustic emission testing.

Incentives in health systems

In a for-profit health system, all kinds of tests will become readily available if there is a market for them. Enthusiasm for breast screening during the 1980s prompted rapid growth in provision in the USA, and competing providers all wanted to ensure they could offer the service. The result was that by 1990 the number of mammography machines in the USA was four times the number actually needed to screen the population. The result, according to an article in the *Annals of Internal Medicine* (Brown *et al.* 1990), was that costs to the consumer were twice as much as in an efficient system, and commercial pressures meant women were encouraged to have mammograms at a younger age and more frequently than the evidence supported.

In health systems depending mainly on public funding, screening may creep in if the initial test is accessible and inexpensive. Less accessible tests tend to wait until there is national or regional endorsement.

There will of course be some provision of the less accessible tests in private clinics, and equipment manufacturers may well install 'free' equipment for the public sector to try and stimulate demand, and they may work with charities and advocacy groups, and run behind-the-scenes campaigns to promote demand, in order to try and secure implementation ahead of evidence. However, where there is a strong tradition of relying on health technology assessment prior to adoption, then these commercial pressures may have relatively small impact. So when, for example, the Forrest Committee recommended in 1986 (Forrest 1986) the introduction of a national programme of mammography screening in the UK, it was possible to plan this completely new service without having to confront any existing entrenched practices.

Implementing from scratch

Imagine you are faced with the task of setting up a new screening programme for your local population. This might be part of a national roll-out or it could be that your locality is a pilot or demonstration project. Some central funding has been earmarked to cover equipment and recruitment of staff to do the screening, but some of the indirect costs will need to be built in to the investment plans for local organizations. The new service is certain to entail some extra work for a range of people.

So the question is, how do you do it?

However difficult the task may seem, it is worth remembering that if the service grows haphazardly it will become a mess, and sorting out a mess is a far greater challenge than setting it up correctly in the first place.

As we explained in Chapter 2, screening must be delivered as a well functioning total system if it is to achieve the best chance of maximum benefit and minimum harm. This system needs to include everything from the identification of those to be invited right through to follow-up after intervention for those found to have a problem.

Your first job is to list all the components of the system and to think through how they will each be planned, funded and managed. Then you have to make it happen.

Often the staff who will be directly involved in the service feel that because they are the experts in bowel cancer, or vascular surgery, or childhood hearing, or antenatal care, then people outside their field, including those in public health, cannot have anything to contribute. If you can encourage them early on to talk to people who have had the experience of establishing screening programmes, albeit in a different field, this can prove very valuable.

On p. 47 in Chapter 2 we briefly introduced the diagram showing the range of components that make up a well ordered programme. The items in the centre are the core activities in the programme, which are likely to be the responsibility of local organizations. The items in the surrounding part of the diagram are essential supporting activities (Fig. 5.1), and it may be that national or regional bodies will look after these aspects.

Now let us think through what each of these components involves, and why it is important.

Aims and objectives

It is essential to have a clear statement of the overall objectives of the programme. If it is a national programme, this should be a national statement. Stakeholders and service users should have input into setting the objectives. Your task is to ensure that the objectives are used to guide local implementation. The objectives must include not only the benefit that screening is aiming to achieve, but also:

+ The need to minimize harm
+ The need to ensure that resources for screening are proportionate, bearing in mind all health needs and the total available resources for healthcare
+ The principles that underpin the information given to participants. In other words, it should be clear that screening is being offered rather than enforced, and that balanced information will be available to enable informed choice (see also Chapter 8, p. 249).

By making explicit the minimization of harm, and the affordability, this can safeguard against the inevitable pressure to maximize sensitivity and to invest ever more for diminishing returns. Pursuing sensitivity irrespective of harmful consequences can lead to escalating overdiagnosis and overtreatment (see Chapter 3, p. 69).

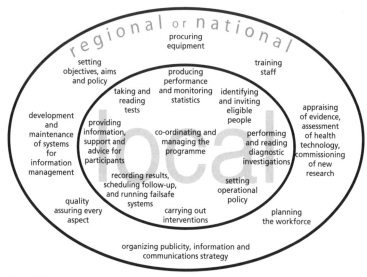

Fig. 5.1 Programme map.

Box 5.1 (p. 132) gives an example of objectives for a screening programme. These objectives were drawn up in 1988. The only significant change between the current 2005 wording and the original 1988 wording is the substitution of 'carry out high quality mammography on those women attending for screening' for the previous wording of 'carry out mammography in a high proportion of those who were invited'. This is because in 1988 there was still an implicit view in the UK (though this was being challenged) that information about screening should be one sided in order to achieve maximum uptake. Now that there is an explicit commitment to giving balanced information (see Chapter 8, p. 249) it is inappropriate to have an objective that implies a requirement to ensure attendance.

The numbers in the flow diagram

When starting a new screening programme, it is helpful to work out the numbers of individuals encountering the different steps in screening and experiencing the various outcomes, for your local population either during a year, or during a 'screening round'. A screening round is the period between screenings, so if screening is two yearly then a

Box 5.1 Aim and objectives of the NHS Breast Screening Programme (NHS Breast Screening Programme 2005)

The aim of the programme is to reduce mortality from breast cancer in the population screened.

The objectives are to:

- Identify and invite eligible women for mammographic screening
- Carry out high quality mammography on those women attending for screening
- Provide services that are acceptable to those who receive them
- Follow-up all women who are referred for further investigations
- Minimise the adverse effects of screening—anxiety, radiation dose and unnecessary investigations
- Diagnose cancers accurately
- Make effective and efficient use of resources for the benefit of the whole population
- Encourage the provision of effective and acceptable treatment that has minimal psychological or functional side effects
- Evaluate the programme regularly and provide feedback to the population served and those working in the programme
- Enable those working in the programme to develop their skills and potential and find fulfilment in their work
- Support audit and research.

round is 2 years. These numbers in the flow diagram provide the 'population pathway' information that we described in Chapter 4 (see p. 117). This can then be used as core information for all involved in planning the service, and for those managing the communication strategy. (We come to an example in the newborn hearing screening case study later in this chapter, see p. 144.)

It is essential to include all the consequences of screening, so that it does not come as a shock later on when staff and the public realize, for example, that interval cancers occur, or miscarriage follows amniocentesis, or complications arise from colonoscopy or tandem mass spectrometry identifies uncertain conditions in newborn babies.

This kind of summary information is starting to be incorporated into information for potential participants in screening. 'Decision aids' are being developed in the form of leaflets, flow diagrams or interactive computer programs that put simple frequencies against the different possible outcomes of screening to help individuals decide what is best for them. Research in this field is relatively new, but growing (O'Connor *et al.* 2001).

Operational policy

A screening programme has to have operational policies to ensure consistent and equitable delivery. Again, these should not be drawn up piecemeal in every different locality, but should be developed, and revised in the light of experience, for the whole programme whether that is regional or national. Your job is to ensure that the policies are understood and are used as the guide for local services, and that feedback is sent to the national or regional people if modifications are needed. Operational policies need to cover a range of issues. Each of the UK NHS cancer screening programmes (NHS Cancer Screening Programmes website) has a long list of publications covering policy and quality standards (for more about quality standards, see Chapter 6). The types of issue covered by operational policies include:

- Who is eligible to be offered screening
- What action should be taken when a test result is equivocal
- Who is responsible for ensuring that investigations, and interventions, are arranged, and for checking they have happened
- Whether future invitations should cease completely for someone who asks not to be screened, and what documentation must be kept to record the person's request
- What risk factors if any qualify an individual for more frequent invitations
- How many times reminders should be sent if a person does not attend for screening
- What action should be taken if a person with an abnormal screening result has moved out of the area

- How the service should deal with requests for screening outside the age range, too frequently or for unusual indications.

System for identifying and inviting

In order to organize a screening programme, it is essential to have a system, preferably computerized, that invites participants, records results, generates reminders for tests, for follow-up, and for failsafe, and produces information about activity that enables the performance of the programme to be monitored and improvements to be planned. This is sometimes referred to as a call and recall system.

Call and recall systems generally encompass the following features:

- There is an up-to-date register of those eligible for screening, based usually on family doctor registrations, or on birth notifications and child health registers.

- The system must be able to cope with patients not registered with a family doctor, of no fixed abode or in prison, in order to ensure that these individuals can be contacted with their results. In the UK there are separate systems for personnel in the armed forces.

- The system must have a means of recording factors that render people ineligible for screening, for example a woman who has had total hysterectomy and has no cervix is no longer eligible for cervical screening.

- The results of screening tests must be recordable by the system, usually linked to an action code.

- The call and recall system needs to be able to exchange data, preferably electronically, with other computer systems that are part of the screening programme. Staff advising the participants need to be able to look up the relevant results. For example, the results of newborn hearing tests need to be electronically transferable to the child health computer system.

- Data protection and confidentiality rules have to be observed, which means having proper security policies and well trained staff. In England and Wales, special exemption from Section 60 of the 2001 Health and Social Care Act has had to be secured at national level simply to allow the cancer screening programmes to continue the service they have been delivering for many years.

- The system must be capable of generating reminders if antici-pated tests or follow-ups have not taken place.

- The system must be capable of recording changes and transmit-ting records appropriately when individuals change name, address, family doctor, administrative area, etc.

- The system must generate accurate annual statistics about the number of people eligible, invited, tested and followed-up.

- The computer should generate letters to those invited, and those at different stages in the screening pathway. These should be clear and informative. Ideally, they should be the same or similar throughout the country. Administrative staff oversee the production of these letters, for many thousands of people, so the letters need to explain who the recipient should contact in order to discuss their results with a clinician. Wording needs great care because the letters are standard, yet the circumstances of those receiving the letters can vary widely. For example, some women receiving a routine invita-tion for mammography screening will have been treated for breast cancer in the past, or may even be terminally ill with breast cancer.

The information technology aspects of these systems may be handled nationally, with standard software issued and updated regularly. Your job is to ensure that those in charge of information technology locally are aware of what needs to happen to establish the call and recall, and that you have sufficient staff locally to manage the system. Staff need to be trained, and to have their work audited regularly. Issues of confidentiality of personal data, and the rules governing exchange of such data need to be included in the training.

Screening tests and diagnostic investigations

Often one of the first decisions locally when starting screening is to work out the optimum setting, size and location for delivery of the screening test, and for subsequent diagnostic investigations. For bowel screening, the test used in the UK is sent by post and performed in the persons own home, cervical screening tests are performed predominantly in family doctor surgeries, and breast screening is done entirely in dedicated breast screening units, some fixed (in buildings) some mobile (in a trailer), serving populations of many hundreds of thousands.

Local implementation needs to examine the options and reach agreement. Key factors to consider include:

- Staff need sufficient workload for maintaining experience and expertise.

- Units should work at full capacity to make efficient use of the fixed cost of equipment and accommodation.

- The geographical location of facilities depends on whether it is only specimens that have to travel, or whether the screened person has to attend in person for a test. Geographical access, particularly for rural populations, is important.

- It is easier to assure the quality of screening if the number of human beings involved is relatively small and if screening is a major part of their job. It is an exceedingly difficult task to guarantee that all the tens of thousands of nurses and doctors who perform cervical screening tests in England have an up-to-date understanding of the programme, are proficient and are giving accurate advice.

- Procurement of equipment for your new screening service is best handled through nationally or regionally led negotiation, involving purchasing, leasing and maintenance agreements.

Interventions

Although treatment services are not technically part of the screening programme, it is nevertheless essential to ensure that everyone with a screen-detected abnormality can receive promptly the interventions they need, performed to a good quality and with proper information and support. This is usually achieved by an expansion in existing treatment facilities. If there are already problems meeting standards for access and quality for those with symptomatic disease then the introduction of screening is likely to highlight the need for more investment, or better management, or both, in the symptomatic service.

Training and workforce development

The mainstay of your screening programme will be the workforce, and it is important to ensure that training, recruitment and staff management arrangements are handled properly.

The work of carrying out and reading screening tests can be repetitive, tiring and demanding. Often when screening first begins the tests are taken and read by highly qualified (and expensive) staff. Once the volume of work grows, then screening is delegated to staff with fewer professional qualifications, trained specifically to meet screening competencies. So in cervical screening in the 1960s experienced doctors read the routine cytology tests. The mainstay of the workforce is now the cytoscreener. Sustaining the workforce can be even more difficult than recruiting staff in the first place. Ways of varying the work so that staff rotate between reading screening tests, entering data, telephone answering and other tasks may help to maximize job satisfaction and minimize fatigue. Involving all grades of staff in annual reviews of the quality of the service, in educational meetings, in quality assurance visits and in activities that bring them in contact with the recipients of screening can help to ensure that all feel valued as essential members of the team.

When implementing new screening programmes it can be highly beneficial to establish designated training centres that provide a model service and that run training programmes for staff visiting from across the region. It is important to make sure that during training the staff are encouraged to voice any concerns that they may have, and to discuss openly the inevitable occurrence of disease in people who have had normal screening results, and other potential harms from screening. Training that brings together, at least for some of the time, staff working in related but physically separated elements of the screening programme helps build recognition of the need for teamwork and good communication across the system.

Communication strategy

Right from the start, you need to make sure that appropriate information is communicated to everyone who needs to know about the screening programme, and that this is done in a clear, consistent, professional and readily understandable way. Most healthcare organizations now have dedicated communications officers, and it is best to enlist their help and draw up a strategy early on. You need to bear in mind the needs of many audiences and stakeholders, for example:

- Senior managers and board members of the organizations who will become responsible for the quality and ongoing funding of the programme.
- Members of the public including those who will and those who will not be eligible for invitation.
- Users of the service, particularly local and national suppor groups, patient organizations and charitable or voluntary organizations that relate to the screening activity. Service users should be involved with the planning of the local service, and the development of information and publicity.
- Health service staff, particularly those who feel their work could be affected, and those who deal with general enquiries from the public. It is important that they learn about the service before it is publicized through local media.
- Neighbouring health service organizations, whose plans will need to dovetail with yours.
- Local media, with great care as to messages and timing so that people are given realistic expectations concerning what can and cannot be achieved by screening, and about when the service will be fully established. If there is confusion or negative publicity it can be very hard to recover from this.

By the time you are close to starting screening you will need to have:

- Easy to read, comprehensive information accessible to all health service staff, particularly those who will have some involvement with patients participating in screening.
- General information for the public.
- Specific information for those eligible in order to help them make up their minds whether to accept their invitation for screening. There need to be versions in different languages, and for people with vision impairment, and with learning difficulties. There needs to be explanation of how people with disability, or any kind of special needs, can access the service.

- Specific information for people who test positive on screening, explaining in some detail what the next steps are and what these involve.

- Specific information for people found, on investigation, to have a confirmed abnormality, explaining in detail what the implications are and what the next steps involve.

- Information for managers, board members, etc. that describes the service, its purpose, its management and co-ordination arrangements, its finances, how performance and quality will be monitored and how any potential quality issues will be dealt with through clear channels of accountability.

Co-ordination and programme management

The different elements that make up a screening programme will not work well together unless specific arrangements are in place to ensure this. There is no ideal blueprint for how this should happen. The task of planning a new service tends to create a strong team spirit and close working relationships. It is very important to formalize ongoing liason arrangements, before the planning and project groups disband. If this is not done, then it is only a matter of time before new members of staff come on the scene, new challenges come along, and it is no longer clear who is in charge of what and who communicates with who. The sense that everyone is part of a well-run system does not last long if people in the different parts no longer know each other and if there is no mutual understanding of what the different elements actually do. Key factors that help to ensure co-ordination are:

- Explicit written arrangements requiring that the different elements of the screening programme work together on matters such as implementing national policy changes, dealing with problems and quality improvement.

- Identification of lead individuals for different elements, identification of a programme co-ordinator, and a requirement to produce an annual report.

- Clarification of the lines of accountability and reporting for each of those lead individuals up to the board and clinical governance directors within their relevant organizations. Without this it is easy for the screening service to be disregarded by senior staff in the organizations that are actually responsible for providing it.

◆ Explicit means of involving service users in monitoring and improving the service. It may be appropriate to have service user representation on the co-ordinating group.

◆ Establishment of a co-ordinating group involving leads for all parts of the system, that meets at least twice a year and is responsible for overseeing quality assurance information, hosting quality assurance visits, maintaining up-to-date written local policy statements, carrying out forward planning and producing the annual reports.

◆ Involvement of service commissioners (those who plan and fund services) as part of the co-ordinating group; without this, problems and funding needs within the programme can easily be overlooked because resources for screening are often the lowest priority within a busy hospital.

As well as co-ordination within each local programme, there needs to be co-ordination at national level. For many programmes, a regional sense of identity can also be helpful, particularly relating to quality assurance systems and training centres.

Quality management systems

Every screening programme needs an explicit system for:

◆ Setting evidence-based measures and standards that match the programme's objectives

◆ Supporting all staff in achieving good quality

◆ Measuring performance against the standards

◆ Ensuring that appropriate action is taken where standards are neither met nor improving.

The main tasks when starting a new screening programme are to set objectives and standards, and to establish systems for achieving them, and for monitoring performance and ensuring that action is taken where necessary. National, regional and local elements all play a role, and the job of the local public health practitioner is likely to relate mostly to ensuring that:

◆ annual information is available

◆ is scrutinized and

- that any problems are brought to the attention of those with responsibility for, and the power to rectify them.

Chapter 6 explains how quality assurance processes began, and how they work within a screening programme.

Research and development

Even when a new screening programme is just being established, it is important to anticipate and manage future changes in technology, in understanding of the disease, and in the available interventions. Appropriate research should be commissioned nationally, and the results of research should feed into policy setting and practice. This relates not just to technology for testing and treatment, but also to research aimed at finding better ways of training and using the workforce, and at bringing improvements in information giving to aid public understanding and to support participants.

Case 5.1 Case study—a pilot site for newborn hearing screening

Your district has just been selected as a national pilot site for newborn hearing screening. An e-mail from the head of your employing organization asks you to take a lead role in getting the pilot established.

How do you go about it?

By and large this is a question of project management. You already have a full workload and the screening service needs some dedicated project management, perhaps a day or two per week for 6 months, to get everything organized. So your first tasks are probably to convene a working group, to persuade your bosses that some project management help is essential, and to write a job description and recruit someone. This maybe an existing member of staff who alters their duties for a while, but it is important to be clear about accountability and time scales.

The next task is for the working group to draw up a work programme (a fancy name for a 'to do' list), and to identify who needs

> **Case 5.1 Case study—a pilot site for newborn hearing screening** *(cont.)*
>
> to be involved in the various tasks. It will probably be beneficial to set up subgroups for the main strands of work. Your role is likely to relate to helping and advising the project manager, assembling information about your population and the size of the screening task, and maintaining a general overview since everyone else is focused on their individual elements.
>
> Table 5.1 shows some of the main items that will be on the 'to do' list for your working group as you start the task of getting newborn hearing screening up and running on your patch. In this example, we are assuming that you have the benefit of a national implementation team that is responsible for overall policy and that is supporting the pilot sites. Against each item we have added comments based on the actual experience of establishing the newborn hearing pilots.

Lessons learned

If you ask the following question of people who have set up screening:

> looking back, what are the key bits of advice you would want to give to someone else starting out on a similar venture?

the kind of answers you get are:

> we just had absolutely no idea how much work would be involved, we thought it would be so simple, there's more to a screening programme than meets the eye.
>
> you have to have dedicated time from someone with good project management skills and with a technical grasp of the tests and clinical issues.
>
> you have to get the support of senior clinicians, particularly nursing staff, and a senior manager in each participating organization. Without this you cannot get front-line staff to co-operate with you to get the service up and running.
>
> there are so many different people—staff and service users—who need to understand the screening service and what it is for. Getting these messages communicated right is essential for getting the service running properly.

Table 5.1 Implementing newborn hearing screening

Item	Comment in the light of experience
Defining the objectives	
The National Implementation Team has already worked with the National Association of Parents of Deaf Children to define the overall aim as follows: 'To enable high quality parent-child interaction in the first months of life for all children, to empower parents of hearing impaired children concerning communication options, and to put in place an evaluative culture of service provision'. The local task is to ensure that everyone, including the parents being offered screening, understands the purpose of the screening service.	The aim and objectives are important. The aim is not just to identify deaf children, but to avoid the lost opportunity for best parent–child interaction that can come if there is a long delay in recognizing hearing impairment. If screening is done badly, or if parents are not supported, you will fail this objective. The objectives also make it clear that treatment with hearing aids or implants, is not the only way of enabling a deaf child to communicate. The parents may choose sign language as the preferred means of developing their child's communication skills. This is why the objectives say 'to empower parents...' and they do not say 'to ensure that all deaf children receive hearing aids or implants'.
The numbers in the flow diagram	
Drawing up the numbers helps to clarify the screening system and the workload involved. It was not easy to find a simple summary of the numbers so we asked for help from the national implementation team (Lindsay Kimm and Adrian Davis personal communication). The result is shown in Fig. 5.2. We have shown the numbers deriving from 100 000 newborn babies in order to avoid having lots of decimal places, although most local services would be dealing with a far smaller population. There are differing degrees of hearing impairment and the numbers in the figure, 151 with bilateral, 83 with unilateral, relate to moderate or worse. Some of the detected babies would have been promptly diagnosed	The newborn hearing screening pilots found that the follow-up work needed for uncertain results was around double the need predicted from research. This very often happens once you screen a real population. It seems to be partly due to the self-selection of participants in research, and partly because uncertain categories of disease expand once you are screening for real and are responsible for long-term outcomes in your participants.

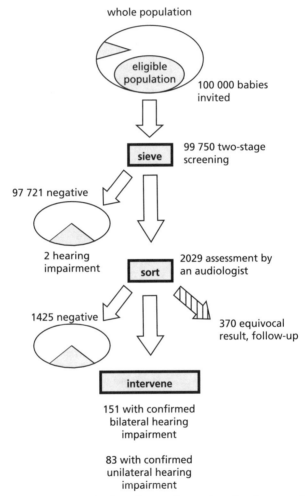

Fig. 5.2 The numbers in the flow diagram for newborn hearing screening.

Table 5.1 (continued) Implementing newborn hearing screening

Item	Comment in the light of experience
even without screening so the programme gives them no real improvement, but we have not attempted to subdivide the numbers in the intervention group according to outcome. Overdiagnosis should be non-existent, although screening does identify some babies with uncertain impairments often accompanied by other problems too. Adverse effects from intervention will arise, but rarely. A very small number of babies, 2 per 100 000, are undetected and are diagnosed later. Parents and staff need to be aware this is a possibility. Similarly some babies and infants will move into the area from places without screening.	
Operational policy Your task will be to take the recommendations in the national implementation team workbook and apply these to your local situation. Some things may need local decision, for example whether to offer screening to babies born in local hospitals but resident in distant districts (you probably will offer it). Other things may include decisions about the balance of hospital versus community testing, and how to do 'catch-up' screening for the babies who were missed during their first month of life (the first month is the ideal time to screen because the baby is calmer, sleeps more, and is less likely to have contracted an upper respiratory tract infection).	It is likely that some operational policy issues will not yet have been anticipated, and one of the tasks of pilot sites is to help develop workable rules, for example over what to do when babies move in or out of the area, what to do about uncertain results, or what to do when there is non-attendance for appointments.

Table 5.1 (continued) Implementing newborn hearing screening

Item	Comment in the light of experience
Call and recall	
Your job is to put into practice whatever the national system is. This should record results, schedule appointments and produce reports of programme performance. This is likely to mean working with a key contact for your local child health computer system, and for each of the information management and technology (IM&T) departments for the hospitals with maternity units. An IM&T subgroup will be essential from the outset, with support from someone senior in this field.	In the local pilot that we used as our model for this case study, the IM&T aspects were quite problematic. All sorts of teething problems emerged when the ready-made software was used, and a paper system had to be used to run the screening programme. Problems of this nature are not uncommon, and thorough testing of screening information systems is essential before they go live. Even for established screening programmes, the development and maintenance of IM&T systems is a major task and a major expense.
Tests and investigations	
You will need to define what tests and investigations are to be used when. You will need to obtain the necessary equipment, and define the procedures for checking and maintenance so as to ensure proper accuracy. Two different types of testing machine are needed. One is the automated otoacoustic screen (AOAE), the other is the automated auditory brainstem response screen (AABR).	The pilots discovered that an average local programme screening about 5000 newborn babies annually needs around five AOAE kits and three AABR kits. Problems with the equipment were very frequent during the pilot, and much time was spent contacting manufacturers and trying to get problems sorted out. This is not unusual. The technology tends to evolve rapidly as it gains widespread use.
Treatment	
Your task is to ensure that timely, appropriate, family-centred intervention is available for each case where hearing impairment is identified. Proper support and advice must also be available for the parents of children with uncertain results needing follow-up. In theory, the workload for audiology departments is not increased since the two babies per thousand (approximately) who have sensori-neural hearing	In practice, the audiology service has extra work during the first 2 years of screening because there is overlap whilst the babies born before the start of the pilot receive distraction test screening. It is important that the service supports and provides early advice to the screeners if they are asked a clinical question by parents. Ideally, the service capacity and the demand can be analysed and managed, and measures should be taken to prevent inappropriate, or lesser

Table 5.1 (continued) Implementing newborn hearing screening

Item	Comment in the light of experience
impairment are only being identified earliar. Also, referrals for temporary conductive hearing loss should be less once the distraction test screening performed at 2 years of age is phased out.	priority work that may burden the audiology service (e.g. referrals by school nurses in children where there are no concerns about language development).

Training and workforce development

You need to recruit and train a team of newborn hearing screeners. This is a relatively new job, and does not yet have a recognized pay scale. Around one whole-time equivalent screener is needed for every 1250 annual births. Many screeners work part time so you are likely to have up to 15 staff for a programme with 10 000 annual births. The National Implementation Team will provide the training. Once the screeners have started, they will still need supervision, support and ongoing training.	Recruitment is often best through adverts in local newspapers. Screeners often find the job repetitive and demoralizing unless they feel valued as part of a team, so a supportive manager for your screeners is important. The pilot sites found that a great deal of work was needed with midwives and ward staff to raise their awareness of the role of screeners. Without this the screeners were made to feel that they were a bit of a nuisance, and it was not easy for them to get time with the babies when they were calm or sleeping.

Communication strategy

You have to make sure that everyone who needs to be aware of the local screening programme gets to hear about it in an appropriate way. Your task is made easier by the fact that there are ready-made national leaflets and a web site, and there are well-established support groups for parents of deaf children. There is nevertheless a lot to do to make sure everyone is informed locally, and help from a trained communications person can make a big difference. The first step is to list all the target audiences, define what key messages you have to convey, and work out the best means of reaching each audience. This forms	One effective method of getting basic information across to staff at all levels is to prepare a couple of paragraphs about the screening programme, in very plain English, and use the existing channels of communication to organize inclusion in staff newsletters for all local health, social care and educational organizations. Make sure to include a contact source for further information. As well as giving information through antenatal clinics, it is worth reaching the general public by issuing a press release for local news contacts. Timing is important; you must not have your press coverage too early or else the public may expect the service to be fully established before it actually is.

Table 5.1 (continued) Implementing newborn hearing screening

Item	Comment in the light of experience
your strategy, then you have to make it happen. Face to face training sessions, with help from parents who have received the service, are the best way of explaining the service to staff such as midwives and health visitors whose direct co-operation will be needed.	A critically important task is to make sure that director level staff in the local healthcare organizations are supportive of the service. Unless they understand the benefits, and are clear about the resources needed and why, they may feel it is just an added burden. All information must give a balanced explanation of the benefits and the limitations, otherwise the expectations placed on the service become impossible to meet.

Co-ordination and programme management

Screening works well when there are able and committed people who feel responsible for the programme and who are prepared to work across organizational boundaries to solve problems and plan ahead. In a robust programme this is not left to chance. Regional or national directors should make sure that every local programme has leadership, explicit lines of responsibility and adequate resources. When screening starts, you need to devise programme management arrangements that will keep things going even when key staff leave, when ring-fenced resources come to an end or when administrative structures are reorganized.	In our experience, there are two quite simple things that help to keep a local programme from falling apart. One is the requirement to produce an annual report, no matter how short, covering the work of the whole programme. The other is the requirement for a co-ordinating group to meet at least twice a year involving lead individuals from all the separate organizations that play a part in the programme. The main tasks of this group are to ensure that the programme is following national advice and policy, is meeting quality standards and is preparing an annual report. Educational events that involve a wide range of staff involved in the programme can also be very beneficial.

Quality management systems

It is not usually the role of the local service to set quality standards, as these need to be set for the whole programme, which may be national or regional, in order to ensure consistent quality throughout. The local task is to ensure that everyone involved understands the standards,	Examples of quality standards for the newborn hearing pilot are: ♦ The screen-positive babies must all (100 per cent) have their audiological assessment done within 4 weeks of screen completion, unless this is deliberately delayed for diagnostic

Table 5.1 (continued) Implementing newborn hearing screening

Item	Comment in the light of experience
is supported in meeting the standards, that data is collected accurately and outset, and to monitor local performance and take action if standards are not met. Local programmes can also provide valuable feedback to the national team about the usefulness of the standards, and of any practical difficulties in an everyday service setting.	reasons or unless audiology is refused by the parents.efficiently from the ♦ The percentage of screened babies that are referred on for audiological assessment should be no more than 3 per cent—the purpose of this standard is to ensure that local programmes do not 'play safe' and refer far too many babies with all the consequent anxiety and over investigation that this leads to. ♦ There must be a named person with responsibility for co-ordinating the programme for each defined geographical area ♦ Information showing performance against standards for each local programme must be published annually in a report for the region.
Research and development The fact that you have volunteered to be a pilot means that you are contributing to national research and development. Both quantitative and qualitative information about your pilot will be used to inform the subsequent implementation stages.	You will probably receive lots of requests for data, the preparation of which will come on top of everyone's official job descriptions. Staff and service users from your pilot may well be asked to give presentations at conferences, and to give advice to new programmes as they begin.

Creating order out of chaos

All too often screening enters routine practice without a clear policy, without clear objectives or standards, and with no structure for organizing all parts of the screening system as an overall programme. For example, antenatal Down's syndrome screening in the UK came into practice without clear national policy, which meant that the methods, the quality, the staff training and the information for prospective parents varied hugely from place to place. In this situation, participants are not really being offered access to a quality-assured screening programme that definitely achieves more good than harm. Instead they are offered tests, delivered to ill-defined standards, with no system for ensuring that appropriate interventions and support are offered should the results not be normal.

The problems with haphazard screening are:

- Lack of quality standards and training can mean that participants are exposed to harmful practices. For example, amniocentesis may be performed without ultrasound guidance by unskilled staff, thereby putting babies at risk. Screening test results may be so unreliable because of poor practice that invasive diagnostic investigations are done where screen results should have been negative, whilst true cases have negative results and go undetected.

- Without the protection of national guidance, clinicians are likely to err on the side of caution for fear of undetected cases. With cancer screening in particular, this can result in many people being advised to have regular follow-up for even the most minor degree of abnormality. Far from being safe, this increases the medically induced harm from screening.

- Without a failsafe system, the people with screen-detected abnormality may receive no proper investigation and intervention following their abnormal screening result. They may not be aware of the significance of the result, and may not know what help to seek.

- There is likely to be inequity, with the highest risk people being the least likely to access the screening.

- Substantial resources may be used in performing very frequent screening in the lowest risk most affluent groups. Although this may be popular, it compounds health inequalities and it uses excessive resources for small, if any, improvement in public health.

The task you are faced with, as a local public health practitioner, is to turn this mess into a well ordered high quality service that delivers more good than harm for your population at affordable cost. How do you do it?

In theory, the task is similar to the task of implementing from scratch. In practice it feels very different because:

- Most people will not see any problem with the status quo. There are probably no data to show who is and is not being tested, what the outcomes are or what resources are being devoted to the screening. Once you set quality standards and collect data, then the scandals start, but when screening is totally haphazard there is little pressure for change.

- If you try and impose policy and standards, you face problems because people do not like change, you may upset commercial interests and professional and research empires, and hostility arises when you try and share out the resources more fairly.

So the critical steps in sorting out a mess are:

- Demonstrate how and why the existing situation is harmful, dangerous, wasteful and inequitable
- Gain commitment from the most senior levels to sorting out the mess
- Clarify and gain commitment to the public health objectives for the screening programme.

These steps may take years to achieve. Once there is widespread acknowledgment of the problem, and clarity about and commitment to the public health objectives of the programme, it then becomes possible to tackle the tasks already described in this chapter for setting up a well ordered programme. The main differences now are that:

- The task is not about straightforward project management. There are winners and losers, and lots of ways in which people can resist change. It is about change management.

- There are no new resources so you have to change the way existing resources are used, which can be very difficult.

Each screening programme tends to have its own special features, problems and keys to sorting out the mess. Here are some lessons learned from sorting out different programmes in the UK:

- Down's syndrome—take the time and trouble to make sure that everyone is clear on the aim, which is to offer choice to the pregnant woman and her partner, it is not a programme for preventing Down's babies being born.

- Sickle cell anaemia—— the population served by the screening must be involved in decisions about policy and delivery.

- Thalassaemia—cultural factors are very important.

- HIV—you must clarify the aim of screening, who and what it is actually for.

- Ultrasound in pregnancy—a test looking for multiple conditions, but done to give a photograph to the parents, is hard to evaluate and does not clarify decision making for any condition.

- Vision—sometimes the best you can achieve is a reduction in the frequency and the numbers of tests and investigations.

- Chlamydia— traditional screening programmes are not a good model for controlling a communicable disease.

- Breast cancer—at least 5 years is needed to develop a new programme.

- Vascular disease—you must prioritize and keep risks and benefits in proportion, or else everyone will be taking harmful and expensive drugs.

- Diabetic retinopathy—be clear about the boundary between a specific screening programme and good clinical practice.

- Cervical cancer—sorting out a mess is very difficult, so never get into a mess in the first place.

Your greatest strength comes from information and your ability to use it well. Remember that it is more powerful to share with people the facts that made you realize that the screening is a mess than just to tell them your conclusions or your plans for change. Once there is commitment to making changes, then your greatest allies are those staff involved in the screening programme who have already, within their own localities, started trying to deliver the screening as a well ordered system. You need to harness their energy and expertise for devising the policies, standards and training that will create order for the whole programme.

Summary points

If tests are accessible, or if commercial incentives for offering tests are inherent in the healthcare system, then screening will start irrespective of evidence and policy.

A well ordered screening programme that does more good than harm usually requires all of the components shown in Fig. 5.1 (p. 131).

When implementing an entirely new screening programme locally, it is usually advantageous to have someone who can dedicate time, over the course of several months, to managing all the start-up arrangements.

The task of starting a new programme builds team spirit and strong relationships between those working in different parts of the system. This will not necessarily continue once screening is routine, unless specific arrangements are put in place. It helps if there is clarity about lead responsibilities and accountabilities, and if there is a requirement for a co-ordinating group to meet and to produce an annual report.

If screening has grown haphazardly, this will expose the public to direct harm because of unreliable tests, inappropriate and potentially harmful investigations and lack of appropriate follow-up and intervention (too much and too little). There will also be inequity and inefficiency.

To sort out a mess and turn it into a well ordered quality-assured screening system, the first hurdle is to get the problems recognized, as the screening may be popular, the harms unrecognized and the lack of benefit unnoticed. This may take time, but is achieved by documenting the problems and by carefully disseminating this information.

Test yourself

Question one

You need to establish bowel cancer screening for your local population, as part of a new national programme. There will be a regional centre organizing the issuing and reading of tests, and there will be a 'screening unit' in one of your local hospitals where screen-positive individuals will be referred for colonoscopy. Your responsibility as public health lead is to 'commission' the different service components from the relevant providers, through your usual funding and contracting mechanisms, and to ensure that your population is properly served by a high quality and co-ordinated programme. The endoscopy services manager in the local hospital has released one of her staff for 1 day a week to work with you during the implementation phase.

(a) What would be the first thing you would do faced with this task?
  You have decided that you need to convene an Implemention Working Group to get the process started.

(b) Jot down some of the key individuals who you think should be asked to be on the Implementation Group

Question two

In your district, the provision of Down's syndrome screening during pregnancy is very haphazard. Different tests are offered, many women resort to private testing, but few complaints are received and nobody seems to regard the situation as much of a problem or a priority for change. You are aware that some private ultrasound services are referring large numbers of pregnant women for amniocenteses. You also have concerns about the quality of the amniocentesis service, and you have received information that confirms that couples are being given very inaccurate information about risks and benefits. You have raised your concerns with relevant medical directors and senior managers over the course of the past year but your concerns have been ignored and denied. National standards for Down's syndrome screening are in the process of being formulated.

(a) Summarize why these concerns are a public health problem

(b) What might you do to begin to improve matters?

Quality assuring screening programmes

The aim of the chapter

In this chapter we:

- Explain why quality assurance is essential if screening is to do more good than harm

- Describe some of the history and thinking that has shaped approaches to quality in industry and in healthcare, focusing on two founding fathers of quality—W. Edwards Deming, and Avedis Donabedian

- Explain some of the ways of measuring screening quality, setting standards and ensuring standards are met.

Why quality assurance is essential in screening

Once you have been personally involved in screening that has no quality assurance, you are left in no doubt as to its importance. If you run a railway with no timetables, no signals, no staff training, no maintenance and no customer information, then you will fail to get people quickly and safely to their destinations and you are soon likely to be closed down because of deaths and injuries in the crashes that inevitably occur. If you run a screening programme with no evidence, no standards, no training, no safety checks and no support for people with abnormal results or with side effects from intervention, then you are similarly unlikely to meet your aim of improving the public's health and, as with the railway, you will ruin people's lives. The popularity paradox (see Chapter 3, p. 68) means the programme will not be closed down, because people with positive results all believe they owe their lives to the screening even if they are left harmed by side

Box 6.1 Poor quality screening is worse than no screening

If screening is worth doing it is ONLY worth doing if done well. Even evidence-based screening will do harm and little good unless delivered as a quality-assured programme.

effects from pointless intervention. Their gratitude is small comfort to the public health practitioner who can see from the numbers that there is no measurable impact on serious disease, and that people are definitely being harmed. The Hippocratic oath does not have a let out clause saying it is alright as long as you mean well, or as long as the subjects think they have been helped.

There is lots of jargon about quality and how to achieve it, and a growing industry creating theory around the subject. In our view, much of this is fairly irrelevant. It does not matter whether you call something 'quality control', 'quality assurance', 'quality improvement' or 'quality management', or if you add in words such as 'total' or 'continuous'. It is all about doing the right thing right, and this is only possible if you focus on the population's real needs, if you build on and use knowledge, and if there is co-operation between all the people involved in different parts of the service.

Some history

Deming's 14 principles

Deming was an expert on quality control and quality improvement. He had been greatly influenced by one of the founding fathers of quality assurance, Walter Shewhart, an American physicist working at Bell Laboratories who used statistics to measure and then improve industrial quality. During the Second World War, as part of the astonishingly speedy creation of a mass production line for planes and tanks, the War Department created a think-tank to develop and teach quality control at the prestigious private University of Stanford at Palo Alto, California. Deming was a member of this think-tank, but after the war his ideas were largely ignored by American industry. The 1950s was a glorious American decade—American factories

Box 6.2 Quality and the American car industry

The huge black Buick limousine pulled smoothly out of the General Motors' garage in Dearborn, Michigan, and glided homewards towards Motown's exclusive suburb of Grossepoint. It was the early 1960s. Nothing, it seemed, could stop the American miracle epitomized by the relentless growth of the car industry. The executive settled confidently in his comfortable seat. His car was faultless. Everywhere his eyes roamed he saw cars built in Detroit. All Americans bought American cars, or so he thought. But his confidence was based on illusion. Americans in and around Detroit bought American cars because they were employees and received special offers. In the rest of America this did not apply. Not only that, but the quality of his car was also an illusion. Any faults that did appear were identified and dealt with, sometimes without asking, in the executive garage to which the car was driven every day. So the faultlessness of his car was a result not of high quality engineering and production but of a personal fault-finding and correction system.

The American car industry was about to be overtaken. The Japanese car industry, which Detroit assumed produced poor quality goods, was to become the world leader, and David Halberstam's book, *The reckoning* gives a brilliant account of the saga (Halberstam 1986). At the heart of the matter was the change brought about by the Japanese. It was true that they used to produce poor quality goods, but they turned this around by deliberately focusing on quality. What was eventually most irritating to many Americans was that they did so not by looking to any ancient Japanese custom of craftsmanship but by listening to an American called W. Edwards Deming.

produced televisions, refrigerators, cars and many other goods, all for American consumers and without competition; who needed quality assurance? Japan's situation was different. Times were fiercely harsh after the Second World War and the Japanese, with no oil of their own, knew they had to export or remain an impoverished and starving country. Deming was sent to Japan in 1946 by the Economic and

Scientific Section of the War Department to study agricultural production. During this and subsequent visits, his ideas on quality assurance principles made a strong impact on key Japanese figures, and were absorbed and used to create the Japanese industrial miracle of the 1970s and 1980s.

Deming was much more than a statistician. He believed that quality assurance was not just about systems for finding and discarding faulty components. It needed a cultural change, which he defined in his 14 key principles, shown in Table 6.1. This culture change was adopted with enthusiasm throughout Japanese industry.

Table 6.1 Deming's 14 principles of management

1.	Create constancy of purpose.
2.	Adopt the new philosophy. We are in a new economic age. Western management must awaken to the challenge, must learn their responsibilities, and take on leadership for change.
3.	Cease dependence on inspection to achieve quality. Eliminate the need for inspection on a mass basis by creating quality into the product in the first place.
4.	End the practice of awarding business on the basis of price tag.
5.	Improve constantly and forever the system of production and service.
6.	Institute training on the job.
7.	Institute leadership.
8.	Drive out fear so that everyone may work effectively for the company.
9.	Break down barriers between departments.
10.	Eliminate slogans, exhortations and targets for the work force that ask for zero defects.
11a.	Eliminate work quotas on the factory floor. Substitute leadership.
11b.	Eliminate management by objective. Eliminate management by numbers, numerical goals. Substitute leadership.
12a.	Remove barriers that rob the hourly worker of his right to pride of workmanship.
12b.	Remove barriers that rob people in management and in engineering of their right to pride in workmanship.
13.	Institute a vigorous programme of education and self-improvement.
14.	Put everybody in the company to work to accomplish the transformation.

The story is described by Kaoru Ishikawa, son of one of Deming's first champions in Japan, in his book *Total quality control the Japanese way* (Ishikawa 1985).

The validity of Deming's principles will be recognizable to anyone who has been involved in a service that has successfully improved its quality to meet public health goals. For example, if you look back at our case study in Chapter 1 (see p. 19) you will see that before the 1980s the UK cervical screening programme was ignoring virtually all of Deming's principles. There was no clarity of purpose, no leadership, no training, no co-operation between different parts of the system, staff were exhorted to prevent every case by 'doing screening properly' (but they were not told how), and all were fearful of being made a scapegoat for the programme's failings. A few local services instituted leadership and purpose as best they could, but this required the rare and often transient coincidence of senior support, resources and skilled local leadership. It proved impossible with such heavily decentralized arrangements to achieve the required quality. The relaunch of the programme in 1988 created centralization for the task of setting objectives, and overseeing quality. However, the work at the centre was achieved not by a team in Whitehall cut off from what was happening throughout the service. Instead it was achieved by using the knowledge, experience and ideas of everyone working throughout the programme. This approach matches Deming's principles. It also matches the features that James Surowiecki describes as essential for successfully harnessing tacit knowledge within an organization. These ideas are described in Surowiecki's book *The wisdom of crowds. Why the many are smarter than the few* (Surowiecki 2005).

Although the principles of achieving quality are universal, Deming's work focused on industrial and manufacturing processes. In healthcare, it is difficult to translate directly the measures of quality that are useful in an industrial setting. It was the work of an Armenian American, Avedis Donabedian, which shaped much of our current thinking on healthcare quality.

Healthcare quality and Avedis Donabedian

There used to be a widespread view that quality in healthcare coul not be defined or measured. Then, in the 1960s, Professor Avedis Donabedian of the University of Michigan was asked to summarize and analyse the literature on quality assessment for healthcare. In his own words, Donabedian said this took 6 months of steadfast work and at the end of it he was quite unsure if what he had achieved was any good. His publisher was in no doubt, saying 'Man, you've written a classic' and the article published in 1966 in the *Millbank Memorial Fund Quarterly* (Donabedian 1966) set out the now famous classification of methods, using structure, process and outcome.

Donabedian defined quality as the degree to which a service conforms to pre-set standards of goodness. One component of quality is the effectiveness of care, or in other words the degree to which it achieves attainable improvements in health. There are other components too, and all are helpful when drawing up pre-set standards of goodness for a screening programme. Donabedian gave a summary of his seven components in his last book, *An introduction to quality assurance in health care* (Donabedian 2003). We explain the components on p. 161, but first we need to outline an approach to quality assurance in screening.

Applying quality assurance to screening

To tackle the task of quality assuring screening you have to:

- Define the objectives of the programme in a way that encapsulates what a 'good' screening programme will look like. Things that can help are Donabedian's seven components, Deming's principles, and the research experience and results that provided evidence for the programme in the first place.

- Devise ways of measuring quality that will ensure these objectives are met.

- Set standards for each measurement; this is a subjectively chosen level that you want the programme to achieve.

- Give responsibility to the local programmes for monitoring how well they are doing in meeting the standards, and for working to improve quality to meet the standards.

- Collate information about performance against standards and publish this nationally for all the local programmes.

♦ Provide support mechanisms for overseeing quality and for assisting local programmes with training and quality improvement. One way of doing this is by creating Regional Quality Assurance Teams.

Quality assurance is a dynamic process, and strong communication between local teams and the Regional and National leads will ensure that standards and measures evolve appropriately.

The seven components of quality

Donabedian's seven components of quality are listed below, and for each we give a brief explanation of the relevance for screening.

Efficacy

Efficacy is the ability of the science and technology of healthcare to bring about improvements in health when used under the most favourable circumstance.

This means that it is impossible to devise good quality screening where there is no evidence that the screening does more good than harm. This applies, for example, to some new uses of tandem mass spectrometry in newborn babies, and to prostate cancer screening. So a starting point for quality screening is to base your policy on valid evidence from high quality research (see Chapter 4 for more about what constitutes valid evidence, and Chapter 8 for more about policy making.)

Effectiveness

Effectiveness is the degree to which attainable improvements in health, the efficacy, are, in fact, realized.

This means that you have to take account of what can actually be achieved in the everyday reality of your health system, and for a whole population, rather than in a research setting dealing only with consenting research subjects. Your quality standards must be deliverable 'on a wet Wednesday in Middlesborough'—or in any ordinary place staffed by ordinary people and including deprived areas in its catchment.

Efficiency

Efficiency is the ability to lower the cost of care without diminishing attainable improvements.

This means that in a good quality programme you use the most efficient way of achieving the outcomes you want, so, for example you make maximal use of the capacity of fixed resources such as X-ray machines, and you streamline all your pathways and processes.

Optimality

Optimality is the balancing of improvements in health against the costs of such improvements.

This means that you cannot ignore the unavoidable economic reality; what you spend on one thing cannot be spent on another. Quality standards in screening must take account of optimality. For example, frequency of testing, addition of new tests, or lowering of thresholds for intervention should only be incorporated if they produce greater health improvement than other alternative ways of using the same resource. For example, guidelines recommending when to treat people with screen-detected risk factors such as raised blood pressure or raised serum cholesterol now mean that as many as 90 per cent of adults over 55 in the USA are defined as 'needing' lifelong treatment for hypertension (Moynihan and Cassels 2005), and even in conservative Britain we are seeing recommendations that could put 25 per cent of 40 to 75 year olds on lifelong statins (Mackenzie *et al.* 2006). The cost-benefit of treating medium risk levels is very poor; side effects are substantial.

Acceptability

Acceptability is conformity to the wishes, desires and expectation of patients and their families.

This means that good quality screening is offered rather than imposed, and that interventions are designed in accordance with the wishes of participants. In newborn hearing screening, for example (see Chapter 5, p. 143), quality standards ensure that parents are involved in choosing how best to manage hearing loss in an infant. Within the deaf community, teaching an infant sign language from an early age may be preferable to surgical intervention using cochlear implants. It can of course be extremely difficult to deliver mass screening in a way that suits every individual. Some people, for example, find it unacceptable to be sent repeated reminders and encouragements to attend screening, whilst others (usually because they have suffered a potentially avoidable condition after not attending) complain they did not receive enough direct encouragement.

Legitimacy

Legitimacy is conformity to social preferences as expressed in ethical principles, values, norms, mores, laws and regulations.

This means, for example, that in a good quality screening programme the testing of pregnant women for Down's syndrome would not take place without first exploring whether the option of termination of the pregnancy would be something that participants might consider.

Equity

Equity is conformity to a principle that determines what is just and fair in the distribution of healthcare and its benefits among members of the population.

This means that a good quality screening programme has to conform with contemporary legal and ethical frameworks that determine what is fair for a given society. So, for example, attempts to make cervical screening more efficient by targeting women at highest risk have never been very successful (Wilkinson *et al.* 1992), because this required the exclusion of women from higher social classes, non-smokers and with few or no sexual partners, and is seen as inequitable. Equity also means that services have to be accessible to all eligible groups. It is no good organizing your written information and your appointments system so that only well educated and well organized people find it possible to use the service. Information and services must be appropriate for all eligible people, including those who cannot read, have disabilities, have specific cultural needs, etc.

All the seven components are important. They recognize that the goal of quality assurance is not pursuit of effectiveness at any cost, if for example this worsens optimality. Similarly, they acknowledge the importance of equity and acceptability.

System design and resources

Like Deming, Donabedian emphasizes that quality is achieved predominantly by the way you design your system, and the resources you put into it, particularly with regard to the training and support you give to staff. It requires a genuine and lasting commitment to quality at all levels within the organization. One element of assuring quality is through performance monitoring and readjustment, but it is a mistake to think that measuring, checking and inspecting are the means of achieving quality. They are only a means of obtaining information which, once interpreted, can lead to action to protect and improve quality. Monitoring works best when performed by committed workers themselves, rather than by external inspectors.

So quality depends on:

+ system design and resources, and

+ monitoring and readjustment.

The evidence upon which a screening programme is based comes from research trials conducted by research workers. Good research workers are obsessional. They prepare and follow a protocol with precision. If a team is involved, all members of the team are taught how to carry out all the procedures in the protocol. The information collected during the course of the project is much more comprehensive and detailed than in routine healthcare. Furthermore, the researchers are usually more committed to the procedure or service they are studying; they have to be to travel through the purgatory of research funding committees, ethics committees and the necessary paraphernalia of modern medical research.

Imagine that a dedicated and committed research team, working to their protocol for a screening programme, obtains a positive result— for example, a 20 per cent reduction in mortality. What are the implications for the whole population if policy makers decide to introduce the programme nationally?

The main problem facing those responsible for implementing the programme is that a service that has been effective when delivered by a committed, atypical, team to 1 per cent of the nation's population now has to be delivered to the other 99 per cent of the population. The research has demonstrated that when delivered to very high standards, screening achieves more good than harm. This is termed the efficacy or, in other words, the effect in the best possible circumstances. However, the person responsible for rolling out a screening programme nationwide wants to know what the effect of the programme will be when delivered in the ordinary service setting. This is the effectiveness, and it is profoundly influenced by how closely the ordinary practitioners can match the quality and attention to detail that the researchers achieved. If they can come close, then the screening will do more good than harm, but if they do not then they may do the opposite.

In order to ensure that the researchers' achievements are matched in the service setting, the programme must devote a percentage of the total resource to specific mechanisms for achieving and monitoring quality. All staff will have to spend some of their time measuring the quality of what they do, carrying out ongoing training, participating in proficiency testing, and participating in annual assessments and quality visits. Funding for Regional Quality Assurance Teams (see p. 173), or equivalent mechanisms appropriate to the particular healthcare system, must be incorporated into the programme costs.

The importance of building quality in from the start

When standards and quality assurance are built in at the start of a screening programme, it ensures that local programmes:

- Are delivered to explicit evidence-based standards and according to specified protocols, by staff with recognized training who have demonstrated their competency, so that the benefits attained in a research setting are actually achieved
- Keep a balance between sensitivity versus specificity, and the resulting human consequences—false alarms and medically induced harm on the one hand, and undetected cases on the other
- Keep a balance between resources invested in the programme and its outputs, thereby avoiding the tendency to chase diminishing returns.

If a screening programme develops haphazardly without consistent quality assurance, those responsible for the quality face problems because of the absence of these controls. For example:

- Lack of specified aims, policies, guidelines and standards for staff training will mean that screening results are unreliable, the next steps are a hit and miss affair, and interventions may be ineffective or bring undue side effects
- Cut-off points for defining abnormal results are likely to have drifted in favour of maximum sensitivity and it can be difficult to reverse this trend and restore specificity

◆ Drift in frequency and age range have probably resulted in highly inefficient use of resources.

So the best way of quality assuring a programme is to build in the quality before the programme even begins, as we described in Chapter 5. If you do not do this, then you end up with a poor quality service, that probably does more harm than good, and you face a mess that needs sorting out (see Chapter 5, p. 149). You have to reverse the practices listed in the bullet points above, and this can be very difficult. For example, the UK Cervical Screening Programme was relaunched with clear standards and quality assurance processes in 1988, but it took until 2003 (NHS Cervical Screening Programme 2003) before the harmful practice of routinely screening under age 25 was stopped. Screening under 25 does more harm than good because trivial abnormalities are very common and cancer is extremely rare. It results in tens of thousands of young women being categorized as abnormal for each one who might possibly be helped. However, years of screening the under 25s, and years of detecting abnormal cell change in the under 25s had convinced many pathologists and gynaecologists that this activity must be a good thing.

Even where staff are supportive of the new changes, you still face the problem that new quality standards expose problems that previously were undocumented. It may be difficult to persuade the media and the general public that identifying and solving these problems represents progress (see also the case history in Chapter 1, p. 19). The headlines are more likely to say 'Scandal of screening blunders' than 'New measures drive up quality'. Very few people understand the difference between screening failures (due to poor quality performance) and screening limitations, and once the media spotlight is turned on a service it is easy for screeners then to be blamed personally for the limitations of screening (undetectable cases, incurable cases, uncertain results) even though they are now performing to a high standard. This creates fear and hostility, and can block attempts to establish quality assurance processes.

This all underlines the need to build quality assurance processes into screening programmes right from the start.

Defining and measuring quality in screening

To help us think about healthcare quality in a manageable way, Donabedian described the now famous categories 'structure', 'process' and 'outcome'. This enables us to devise standards and measures that relate partly to our facilities and resources, partly to the way that we do things and partly to the outcomes we achieve. Some examples, in relation to a screening programme, would be:

Structure: standards relating to the structure of the programme might specify the laboratory facilities, the staffing that we need, the computer system for call and recall, etc.

Process: standards relating to processes might specify the time to be spent explaining options to participants and the key components of the consultation, the processes to be followed for performing and reading tests, the training, proficiency testing and continuing professional development for screening staff, the calibration and quality controls on equipment, the procedures to be offered at the intervention stage, the timeliness of each stage, etc.

Outcome: standards relating to outcomes might specify the detection rate for screen-detected abnormality, the satisfaction of participants, the rate of occurrence of complications, the incidence of undetected cases, the numbers of cases lost to follow-up, the completion rates for treatment in screen-detected cases, the incidence and mortality rate from the condition that screening aims to prevent, etc.

Quality standards based on structure, process, and short-term outcome are essential, because measurement of long-term outcome alone can bring difficulties. For many conditions, the mortality or incidence at national level can be a useful measure, but for a local programme serving a few million total population, the measurement of local incidence and mortality may have little bearing on the quality of the service. This is because:

- Changes in mortality rates are influenced by factors other than service quality, for example changes in the background incidence, geographical variation due to deprivation and risk factors, population movement and uncertain denominators, and ordinary statistical variation due to small numbers.

- Insofar as the local mortality rate is affected by local service quality, this reflects the quality of the service pertaining to several years ago, whereas the person responsible for ensuring and monitoring the programme needs information about the current state of quality.

So outcomes relating to reduction in deaths or serious cases are rarely of direct use in measuring the quality of a local, as opposed to a national, programme.

Ordinary statistical variation also poses problems when measuring quality for a service with relatively small numbers of tests or procedures. Structural standards often specify a minimum number of tests for the individual screener, or a minimum catchment population for a screening unit. This is partly to ensure adequate experience, partly to ensure efficient use of fixed resources such as equipment, but partly also to give adequate statistical power to spot important variation in performance. The more you can centralize processes into the hands of people specializing in that procedure, then the easier it is to measure performance. However, if the population is best served by small local units, and if there are other reasons why generalist staff should maintain screening as part of their responsibilities, this can bring a real dilemma. One way around this is for small units to affiliate with one another and participate in quality assurance processes as a collective. Their combined statistics should give sufficient power to demonstrate good performance across the consortium.

Choosing what to measure

When devising quality measures for screening programmes you have to decide three things; what to measure, how to measure it and how high to set the standard.

The best approach is to take each objective for the screening service, and select relevant structures and processes that can be measured objectively. These measurements can then be used to assess achievement of or progress towards the objective. This way the performance of an individual, a service or a programme can be defined.

+ These *measures* give an objective assessment of what **is** being achieved.

+ A *standard* is a subjective judgement of a level of performance that **could or should** be achieved.

When choosing what to measure, you need to bear in mind the fact that quality measures should:

- Span all seven components of quality (see p. 161) and should cover a mix of structure, process and outcome

- Make sense to the people who deliver the screening; feedback from staff on the validity and usefulness of measures should lead to readjustment where necessary

- Relate to the objectives for the programme (see p. 130); every objective should have one or more criteria that can be used to measure progress towards that objective, or lack of it.

Deciding how to measure

If you can choose quality measures that the participants and the staff recognize as important, and if you can involve staff and participants in their measurement, then you are likely to create a system of quality assurance that genuinely drives improvement. The following case study illustrates this.

Case 6.1 Case study—experience from the cervical screening programme

In one English region, the first attempts to start region-wide quality processes for cervical screening were met with fear and hostility. The Regional Co-ordinator worked at Regional Headquarters, had no direct involvement in screening and was seen as being outside of the programme. He would call meetings of the leads from all the local programmes, but the meetings achieved little and there was obvious mistrust of the process. On one occasion, a local manager walked out mid-meeting because he did not think that information about the services should be shared.

Eventually, the Regional Co-ordinator adopted a different approach.

- A trusted and experienced member of staff who ran the call and recall service for one of the local programmes was employed on secondment by the region to visit all the programmes.

Case 6.1 Case study—experience from the cervical screening programme *(cont.)*

- Chairmanship of the regional meetings was delegated to an experienced and trusted pathologist from one of the local programmes.

- The seconded member of staff produced a confidential report, which was shared amongst all the participating programmes but was not disseminated outside the group. The report set out very clearly what the policy and performance was in each locality.

Once this was done, it was obvious that the similarities between the programmes were far greater than the differences, and that all programmes faced the same kind of problems.

From then on, region-wide meetings were positive and productive, policy and standards were soon uniform, and a real understanding and commitment to a unified approach to improving quality was achieved.

In due course, a quality team was established for the region to assist with regular quality assessments and to help with action to improve standards. A part-time secretary worked solely for the team, but all other members were experienced professionals working in screening, who worked for the quality team for a session a week.

The initial hostility was caused by a number of factors:

- When the first attempts were made at establishing quality measures, there was a prevailing belief (not based on evidence) that every single case of cervical cancer in a screened woman must be someone's fault. There was even a notice on the wall at the Regional Cytology Training Centre saying 'Every case of cervical cancer is preventable if only screening is done properly'.

- Every programme knew that they had such cases (but did not know if others did), so there was a great deal of fear.

- The Regional Co-ordinator was seen as an outsider, someone who did not necessarily understand the difficulties of delivering screening.

- There was a feeling that some programmes thought they were better than others, and were out to prove they were the best.

> **Case 6.1 Case study—experience from the cervical screening programme** *(cont.)*
>
> What made the difference?
>
> ◆ The member of staff seconded to do the initial audit was part of the screening service, and understood that everyone did actually care about quality, provided that this focused on realistic and important standards.
>
> ◆ The individual programme leads started to trust the quality assurance process as being about enabling them to meet achievable standards. It was not about blaming people for failing to do the unachievable (i.e. for failing to prevent absolutely every case).
>
> ◆ Once accurate information, clearly presented, was shared amongst the programmes, then the climate of fear and hostility disappeared, since this had been based on misinformation and rumour.
>
> ◆ The new system enabled the local programmes to co-operate in pushing for better training, for better national policy, for better computer support, etc.

Setting standards

When setting standards, it is always difficult to know how high or low to set them. Everyone wants to be treated by an 'above average surgeon', but about half of any group, by definition, will be below average. One way around this is to define minimum, achievable and optimal standards.

◆ The minimum acceptable standard—if a service is not meeting this then urgent remedial action should be taken.

◆ The achievable standard—this could be set as the level of performance achieved by the top quarter of services. If one quarter of services can achieve a certain performance level, almost all services have the potential to do so. One needs to be careful though about recognizing when good is good enough. Once all services improve to meet the achievable standard, it may be more beneficial to concentrate on quality improvement in a different service, rather than raising this standard up to the new level for the top quartile. Pursuit of excellence is all very well as a slogan, but if it comes at the expense of neglect in other areas of healthcare then universal goodness is preferable.

◆ The optimal standard—the best level of service that can be achieved. Although this is a worthy standard, it is often achieved only by exceptional people and/or in exceptional circumstances. The optimal standard may be regarded by colleagues in other services as atypical and therefore of little use for motivating the majority of service providers.

Deming's principle of 'Improve constantly and forever' is sometimes interpreted very narrowly, as meaning that an individual standard, once achieved, should automatically be raised higher. This ignores the need to look for other aspects of quality that may be more in need of attention, and it ignores the need to pursue efficiency and optimality.

What do quality assurance systems actually consist of?

We have explained why quality assurance is essential, and we have given some pointers as to how to measure quality and set standards. However, what does this mean in practical terms for a public health practitioner with local responsibility for screening?

Precise arrangements vary widely, from country to country, region to region and across different types of screening. There is no 'best structure' as this will depend on the specific screening activity, and on how health services are delivered, managed and funded.

In the UK, we tend to have:

◆ Standards and measures that are applied nationally.

◆ Explicit written agreements about responsibilities, lines of accountability, and about who to turn to for support if standards are not achieved and if action is not being taken to address matters. As a last resort, each organization has a policy on 'whistle-blowing' to protect staff if they draw attention to important quality failures.

- Annual statistical returns from each local programme submitted to the Department of Health and published as a national statistical bulletin. This means that anyone can look up the performance for every local programme.

- Regional Training Centres specific to each programme.

- Proficiency testing programmes that screeners have to participate in regularly.

- External quality assurance schemes that measure the consistency and reliability of test performance.

- Quality Assurance Teams specific to each programme, i.e. breast cancer screening, Down's screening, etc., and serving a region. The team assists all local programmes in achieving the necessary standards, and monitors performance against a range of measures, leading to recommendations, with deadlines for achievement. The teams usually have one or two permanently employed administrative staff, but the professional members work in local screening programmes and are employed on secondment for around half day a week to work for the Regional Team.

- Annual Reports produced by the Regional Quality Assurance Teams, based on a rolling schedule of visits supplemented by annual statistical returns and questionnaires. The visits are constructive rather than inquisitorial, and examine all aspects of the service including the strength of the communication and relationships between the elements.

In addition, as in all countries, there are regulatory processes such as the Clinical Pathology Accreditation UK system for laboratories (CPA UK), again requiring detailed visits and submission of evidence of good practice. In contrast to these regulatory mechanisms, the role of the screening Quality Assurance Teams tends to be far more supportive, and involves more direct assistance with achieving improvements in quality.

So a starting point for a public health practitioner taking on new responsibility for a service would be to study the most recent report from the Regional Quality Assurance Team, study the national statistics (an annual National Bulletin is published by the Office for National Statistics, for each national screening programme, giving performance figures for every laboratory and locality), study the national standards and arrange to meet with service leads to build up a complete picture of actions needed to maintain all aspects of necessary service quality. Many quality failures that do occur are a result of poor communication between the different parts of the system, or arise because individual elements become isolated with the result that problems are ignored. It is the job of the local public health practitioner to maintain an overview of quality for the whole system and thereby prevent such failures from occurring.

Summary points

If screening is delivered badly it will do more harm than good, even where there is sound evidence that in a research setting it does more good than harm.

To make sure screening is not delivered badly, you need to design the system and the resources so that quality is a priority, and you need to measure quality so that adjustments can be made where necessary.

Without quality assurance, screening results are unreliable, the next steps are a hit and miss affair and interventions may be at best ineffective and at worst damaging.

Without quality assurance there is no control mechanism for ensuring a balance between good and harm, and for maintaining efficiency and optimality. Sensitivity tends to be pursued exclusively irrespective of harm and cost, and extra resources are invested to pursue narrower and narrower goals regardless of whether this is the best use of these resources.

Quality is achieved by training, motivating and rewarding the staff who deliver the service, and by involving them in measurement of important, realistic and achievable quality standards.

The quality measures for screening should relate to the programme's objectives, cover structure, process and outcome, and take account of all seven of Donabedian's components of quality in healthcare.

A standard is a subjective judgement of a level of performance that could or should be achieved. It is useful to set both minimum

Summary points *(cont.)*

levels and achievable levels. The minimum standard is a level where if it is not met the service needs investigating. The achievable standard is a level you believe all programmes could reach, and it may be set by choosing the level attained initially by the top quarter of services.

As quality improves and all services achieve what previously was achieved only by the top quartile, then it is probably more important to turn to other areas that need quality improvement rather than requiring ever higher standards in certain narrow areas.

Test yourself

Question one

A programme to offer sickle cell and thalassaemia screening during pregnancy is drawing up its quality standards and measures.

Sickle cell and thalassaemia are groups of inherited disorders affecting the haemoglobin in red blood cells. The purpose of offering screening for pregnant women is:

♦ To identify if the mother is carrying a gene that could mean the baby being affected. If the mother is identified as a carrier, then the next step is to offer testing to the father. If the father is a carrier too, then the pregnancy is deemed 'high risk'—meaning a risk of around one in four of having an affected baby. The couple is then offered prenatal diagnostic testing for the foetus. If the foetus is affected, then the couple is supported in making an informed choice about termination, or continuing with the pregnancy. Testing of newborn babies identified as at risk may also be needed.

From this you can see that the programme deals with difficult and sensitive issues, and that informed choice is a key underlying feature. It can be a real challenge to ensure that all the steps, involving offering and explaining testing, performing the tests, communicating the results and providing skilled counselling, are taken swiftly to enable the option of early termination for a seriously affected pregnancy.

Listed below are five of the programme's objectives A–E. Below that we have listed five quality criteria F–J relating to each of the five objectives, but these are not in the same order as the objectives. Below that are five achievable standards K–O relating to each of the five objectives, but again these are not in order. Your task is to match up, for each objective, the criterion and the standard that go with it.

Five objectives

A. To ensure screening tests are offered by 8–10 weeks of pregnancy by primary care (i.e. the family doctor service) or the maternity services.

B. To process and report results of screening in a timely manner.

C. To provide timely expert counselling for women/couples identified with 'high risk' pregnancies.

D. To minimize the adverse effects of screening—including anxiety, misunderstanding, failure to communicate results, inaccurate information, unnecessary investigation and follow-up, and inappropriate disclosure of information.

E. To diagnose specified conditions accurately where prenatal diagnosis is undertaken.

Five criteria

F. Laboratory frequency of sample analysis should be at least twice weekly, and carrier results plus advice on the result should be reported to the woman tested, or the partner if tested, within 5 days of the laboratory report.

G. National prenatal diagnostic testing processes, and chorionic villus sampling processes should be followed, critical events should be reported and monitored, sensitivity and specificity for prenatal diagnosis compared with newborn diagnosis should be recorded for each laboratory.

H. The family doctor service or maternity service should offer screening to all pregnant women presenting to the services, by week 10 of pregnancy.

I. Women and partners with identified 'high risk' pregnancies should be counselled by counsellors (or other personnel) with appropriate training and skills.

J. There should be effective communication of all antenatal screening results in a standard and easy to understand format, to relevant professionals including the woman's health visitor and her family doctor.

Five achievable standards

K. Ninety-five per cent of units to have PEGASUS- (this is a national network providing recognized training) trained counsellors for providing counselling for couples with 'high risk' pregnancies.

L. Ninety-nine per cent sensitivity and specificity, for prenatal compared with newborn diagnosis, achieved for all pregnancies where prenatal diagnosis is undertaken as part of the programme.

M. Seventy-five per cent of women to have an offer of screening by 10 weeks of pregnancy, evidenced by a record in the notes.

N. Ninety-five per cent of units to be performing testing at least twice weekly, and 90 per cent of results to be provided verbally and in writing to women, or their partner if tested, within 5 days, recorded by date of dispatch of letter.

O. Eighty-five per cent of maternity units to be reporting screening results in a standard format to the patient's family doctor and health visitor.

Question two

For the programme objectives in question one, can you give an example of a quality failing that could happen if this objective is not met, but that should not happen if the quality assurances are successfully in place. We give you an example using objective A, so you need to complete examples for B, C, D and E.

For example, for objective A (offering screening to all by 10 weeks of pregnancy), an example would be:

A woman reaches 30 weeks in her pregnancy then asks about thalassaemia screening. She had assumed that tests must have been done because she has Greek grandparents and is therefore more likely to be a carrier than someone with white British family origins. She had not been offered the tests in early pregnancy, and it is now too late to consider screening and possible termination if her baby has a serious condition.

Chapter 7

Day to day management of screening for public health practitioners and programme managers

The aim of the chapter

After reading this chapter, you should have an appreciation of some of the main issues that public health practitioners regularly deal with in screening, and how to approach them.

It might be easy to assume that public health involvement is only needed locally when implementing a new programme; then, once the programme is started, it will tick over smoothly for ever and a day. Evidence and policy making are matters for central attention, so local practitioners surely play no role. In practice, life is not like this, the inboxes of health service managers everywhere are full of problems related to screening. To sort out these problems effectively needs not only management skills, but also an understanding of screening programmes. Typical problems are:

- Preventing screening from starting when there is no sound evidence base. This might be before there is certain evidence, where research trials are therefore needed or are in progress but not yet complete, or it may be that evidence does exist showing either that harm exceeds benefit, or that the cost of the screening is excessive and resources should be used for other needs.

- Dealing with provision of screening where there is no quality assurance, or no evidence base, or both. Provision of this kind of screening will be causing more harm than good. Sometimes this relates to screening where there is good evidence, so the problem is how to sort out the mess (this is dealt with in Chapter 5, see p. 149). Sometimes it relates to screening with no good evidence, so the problem is how to persuade professionals to stop providing it, and people to stop wanting it.

♦ Implementing policy changes to, or solving problems within, established evidence-based quality-assured programmes.

♦ Concerns about commercially driven screening where there is lack of evidence, lack of consumer information, or no provision of investigations or interventions or support for people with positive screening test results.

♦ Screening and the law.

The task for the local practitioner is partly to deal with what is happening on your patch, and partly to communicate with colleagues at the regional or national tier, for example to request more research, or request adjustments to policy, or request clearer or stronger guidance confirming what is and is not recommended and why.

The essential challenge inherent in the first two problems listed above is how to deal with demand for, or provision of, screening that you believe will have a harmful impact on your local population, because of either direct harm, diversion of resources or lost opportunity for beneficial research. The first part of this chapter therefore explains ways of controlling demand for, or provision of, inappropriate screening. We recognize that sometimes there can be a difference of interpretation about what is appropriate and what is inappropriate screening, and that everyone will not always agree with national policy. There may, for example, be a frustratingly long time lag between the assembly of evidence for a new programme, and the point where a properly resourced quality-assured programme can be implemented. There may also be circumstances where you disagree with national policy to introduce screening because locally you feel that other neglected service improvements are a higher priority for investment. You can communicate your concerns, but if the national programme goes ahead then your population is best served by your efforts to ensure that this is delivered to a high quality. Also, if national policy is not to screen, then your population is best served by the avoidance of haphazard testing. The threshold at which you get directly involved in discouraging, stopping and reversing harmful screening may vary from circumstance to circumstance. The skills involved are nevertheless an essential competence for public health practitioners, whatever the debate about precisely when they should be applied.

The second section of the chapter deals with the skills needed for handling day to day issues in established screening programmes, the third deals with commercial sector problems, and the fourth with screening and the law.

Dealing with any of these matters can involve using the media. Even if you are used to producing press releases and being interviewed, there are still some nasty pitfalls where screening is concerned. The final section of the chapter therefore gives some advice about how to cope when the media spotlight turns on screening.

Coping with demand for, or provision of, inappropriate screening

These problems can come in many guises. For example, you may be faced with:

- Concerns about the harm, and the diversion of resources, from 'routine' use of simple tests. For example, routine dipstick urine testing, which detects microscopic amounts of blood in the urine, leads to around 500 people needing a hospital investigation known as cystoscopy, for each one case where underlying disease is actually found. Even then there is no evidence that outcome is any better than if the diagnosis was made once the condition was symptomatic (Laitner 2002)

- Full-blown local campaigns, with mass media coverage, calling for annual cervical screening or routine prostate-specific antigen (PSA) screening for all men

- A mobile computerized tomography (CT) scanner unit proposing to offer, and advertise, whole-body screening from a site in the main car park of your local hospital. This screening is of no benefit and finds numerous X-ray shadows that then need highly invasive investigations in order to rule out serious illness (US Food and Drug Administration 2005).

In the rest of this book, we have explained the reasons why it is important to manage and control these demands. The reasons are:

- To safeguard the public from harmful consequences of screening for which there is no evidence that benefit exceeds harm
- To avoid diversion of resources away from valuable health service provision
- To allow the opportunity for well conducted randomized controlled trials where the prospect of benefit looks promising.

So the question we need to focus on here is not whether to control inappropriate screening, but how to do it.

The key steps in controlling demand for haphazard or non-evidence-based screening are:

- Understand why people want the screening
- Acknowledge the reasons why people want it
- Assemble and communicate evidence and information about the consequences screening is likely to bring, and about other possible approaches to helping the problem (e.g. primary prevention, improved diagnostic and treatment facilities)
- Introduce specific policy measures to control the screening.

Understanding why people want screening

First you need to find out and understand the reasons why people — public and professionals—are asking for or are already doing the screening. The best way of doing this is by going and listening to them, not with the aim of telling them they are wrong and misguided, but just to listen and understand. The kinds of reasons that come up are:

- Someone close to them is affected by the disease and they want to do something to ensure that others do not suffer in the same way
- They have learned that elsewhere (the USA, other parts of Europe, or privately) screening is offered
- The tests seem simple and cheap
- People who have been screened speak very positively about it, either because they were reassured or because they feel they owe their life to early detection

- Not enough is spent on the disease, and screening is a way of demonstrating commitment to the problem
- Intuitively they feel that screening must save money
- Screening will raise the profile of the disease and improve awareness and understanding
- Magazine or newspaper articles say that screening should be offered
- Screening will give an opportunity for giving advice about personal behaviour change that may reduce risk
- 'Evidence' in the form of case reports, uncontrolled studies or poorly conducted case–control comparisons (see Chapter 4 for explanation of why these are not good evidence) has convinced them that screening will be beneficial.

Acknowledging the reasons for people wanting screening

If your efforts at controlling inappropriate screening are to have any long-term influence, as opposed to fending off pressure in the short term only for it to re-emerge probably more strongly soon after, then you need to try and work with the people wanting screening. You need to demonstrate that you have listened to and understood their reasons, and that you share their overall aim of improving the lot of people suffering from the disease in question. Your disagreement with them is only about the means, not the ends. If you can work with them on implementing improvements to primary prevention and treatment services, and on lobbying for high quality research on screening, then they may become your allies in controlling haphazard demand for screening until such a time as a national high quality screening programme becomes the right thing to do. In our experience, this approach is successful when the pressure for screening is driven by a genuine desire to do what is best for the disease in question.

Sometimes the individual or group is intent on getting screening introduced irrespective of the consequences. There may be commercial reasons, or a research empire to build. It may be a matter of personal pride—they said they would get it introduced and so they will. In our experience, it is very rare for the public to lobby for screening unless there are clinicians somewhere telling them that this is something they should campaign for. Sometimes the justifications for screening are based on wishful thinking, and sometimes on the right to know. Studies that have asked members of the public whether they think screening should be provided even if it is known to do no good find that many people say it should be provided (Peticolas 2003; Schwartz *et al.* 2004). Conveying the concepts of evidence of harm and diversion of resources is a real challenge after a century of misinformation, especially whilst health professionals—for whatever motivations—are still recommending unproven screening. The values and beliefs held by members of society have a profound influence, and we explore their impact on policy in Chapter 8 (see pp. 231 and 235).

When you meet an impasse, you may have to accept that the lobbying will continue, and your work to safeguard the public from haphazard screening will have to proceed in the face of opposition.

Assembling and communicating evidence and information

Once you have engaged with those doing the testing or the campaigning, or both, and you have properly listened to what they have to say, then you can start to assemble and communicate the information you want to get across. You need to put matters in context by setting out things that can and should be done to improve prevention, treatment and care for the disease in question. Within this context, you need to set out the potential benefits (if any), the potential harms and the resources needed for the screening proposal that they are making. This may be introduction of a new screening programme, or it may be an increase in the intensity (additional tests, frequency or eligibility) of existing screening. You need to include a clear explanation of why the screening proposal is less beneficial than other ways of using equivalent resources. How much time and effort you dedicate to this depends entirely on the problem faced. The effort needed can vary from:

- Sending documentation about the national policy to those who have raised the issue of more or different screening

- Sitting down with an individual clinician and working through the numbers and evidence together

♦ Attending a pressure group meeting, entering into a dialogue with them and, by working together, finding alternative proposals for reducing the burden of disease.

When none of the above makes any difference and you are still faced with strong pressure to allow screening that would significantly damage public health then you will need to take more formal action.

It is important to contact relevant national authorities, and regional officials, so they are aware of the pressures you are facing locally. They may be able to offer you help and support, or they may put you in touch with others who have successfully dealt with similar problems.

You will need to prepare proper briefing papers setting out the relevant background and facts. You may need formal documents for the members of the boards of your local health service organizations, a well-worded press statement and an easy to understand question and answer sheet suitable for members of the public. You need to be prepared to cope with television interviews, live 'phone-ins' on local radio, and perhaps ongoing communication with politicians and others over the course of many months or even years.

Working out who are your key audiences, what are your key messages and what are the best means (e.g. mass media, written information, existing newsletters, face-to-face contact, etc.) will help ensure that the communication is effective. Creative ways of conveying dense statistical information will help get your message across. For example, Fig. 7.1 is one way of illustrating why public health practitioners have serious concerns about routine prostate cancer screening using PSA testing (see also pp. 95, 101, and 236). This figure uses data from a detailed review published in the *Lancet* (Frankel *et al.* 2003). The box represents 10 000 men age 50. The dark area at the bottom represents the 300 men, amongst these 10 000, who will be destined to die from prostate cancer at some stage in the future. Nobody would deny that if there were a safe and efficient means of reducing this number, we would want to do it. The shaded area represents the cumulative total of 4200 men who, if PSA screening testing is carried out regularly in the 10 000, will, over the course of the rest of their lives, be found to have pathologically confirmed localized prostate cancer. All these men will face the prospect of a potentially harmful intervention. Some of

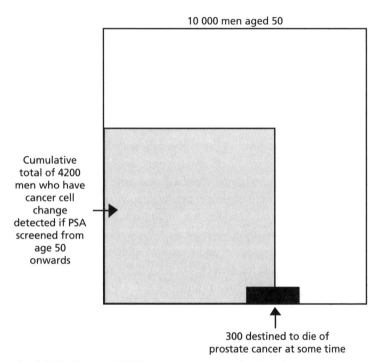

10 000 men aged 50

Cumulative total of 4200 men who have cancer cell change detected if PSA screened from age 50 onwards

300 destined to die of prostate cancer at some time

Fig. 7.1 The human shield in prostate cancer, using data from Frankel *et al.* (2003).

the 300 men destined to die of prostate cancer will be amongst the 4200 with screen-detected prostate abnormality, but we do not know whether screening will stop them getting distant metastatic disease.

The 4200 estimate is based on existing published literature, but in fact the number of men found to have microscopic foci of prostate cancer tissue goes up if you perform biopsies on more men, if you take more pieces of tissue at each biopsy, if you slice the biopsy specimens even thinner for looking at them down the microscope and if you lower the threshold used by pathologists for classifying tissue change as cancer. So, the more you look the more you find, and in fact this elastic number of 4200 could potentially be even higher. It is certain that the vast majority of men with cancer tissue in their prostate glands will never suffer a problem as a result of it, unless that is they are screened and suffer incontinence, impotence or even worse side effects from the cancer treatment.

So, even if all the men with detectable cell changes in their prostates are identified and treated, there is no knowing what change this makes in the long term to the men who are destined to die of their cancer. The dilemma can be likened to the practice of placing innocent civilians, or hostages, as a 'human shield' in military installations targeted for enemy bombing. The men with inconsequential cancers are like a human shield; they have to suffer damage with no benefit if we are even to try and help the cancers that might prove fatal.

Introducing control measures to ensure policy is followed

Sometimes it is both necessary and possible to introduce measures that ensure policy is adhered to. For example, a radiology department, with backing from the hospital board and the relevant authorities that commission services for the population, may issue a clear policy stating that it will not accept routine requests for dual-energy X-ray absorption (DXA) scans in people without a clinical reason for doing the test. A mammography unit can opt to do no routine mammography in women under 50. Laboratories can have a policy of returning to the sender any cervical cytology tests received for women under 25 or for women who have had a routine normal result within the preceding 33 months (National Audit Office 1998).

Restrictions on what is available are commonplace and implicit within health services. In the commercial sector, the restrictions are based on ability to pay. If you want whole-body CT and you can pay for it, then you can have it. If you want your hip replacement operation next week and you cannot pay for it, then you cannot have it. It is not for the commercial provider to worry about what is an efficient or fair use of resources. Within public sector health services, restrictions are based on principles of equity and efficiency. In the UK National Health Service for example, we would not expect to do an exercise electrocardiogram or a magnetic resonance scan on a healthy person even if the person requested it. Efficiency and fair access for all are founding principles of the service (The National Health Service Act 1946), and are reflected in General Medical Council guidance to doctors (General Medical Council 2006). People accept restrictions on what is available because they are used to a collective system of state provision, that limits unfettered access for an individual, in order to achieve fair access for all and best value for public spending. What binds the system together is the indirect benefit for everyone from knowing they live in a society that provides care and treatment for all citizens according to need rather than income.

It is when restrictions seem to reduce or stop what was previously available that we run into trouble. For example, consider town A and town B, both part of a national cervical screening programme where the policy is to screen three yearly from age 25 to 49, and five yearly from 50 to 65. Town A introduced a send-back policy many years ago with the result that no screening tests are carried out more frequently than the policy dictates. To the sample takers and the women in town A this is a matter of course, it is seen as normal. Town B has not introduced send-back, and rivalry between the family doctor services and the local family planning clinics has meant that each offers screening two yearly, and from age 15 in the hope of attracting more clients. Staff and women in town B see this as normal, whereas the staff from town A are astonished at this inefficient (two yearly) and harmful (screening teenagers) practice. If a send-back policy is proposed for town B, it will be seen as denying people access that they previously had. Yet even in town B nobody questions the fact that breast screening more frequently than three yearly can only be obtained by paying privately, or that ultrasound, whole-body CT or electrocardiograms are not available on request for people without a clinical diagnostic need.

So introducing restrictions to control inappropriate screening has to be done in a carefully planned way so that people can see the reasons for it. As a general rule, the following factors are important:

- Plan the controls as early as possible rather than letting inappropriate screening grow and become accepted as 'routine'.
- Involve key stakeholders (e.g. family doctors, laboratory staff, service users, hospital clinicians and managers) in the process of planning the control mechanisms and their introduction.
- Assemble clear information that sets out what the policy is and why.
- Disseminate this information to all key stakeholders and make it available on the web. Do not forget to include senior staff such as top managers and board members, even if the issue seems relatively small. If they are not briefed, then it only takes one phone call from an influential lay person who feels upset by the apparent

restrictions to make your top team feel very vulnerable. Keep national and regional contacts informed too.

♦ Give plenty of advance warning of the date from which the controls will come into effect so that people have time to get used to the idea.

♦ Include names and contact details of the staff who can answer queries. This way you are making it plain that you believe in the policy, its not just about cost-cutting and you are not hiding behind bureaucracy.

♦ At all stages try and put yourself in the shoes of someone who might expect to request a test. Think about, if you were them, what factors would make you feel that the restriction was fairly thought through and reasonably implemented.

♦ Be prepared to deal with questions from politicians if members of the public or disgruntled professionals contact them. Be in a position to send a sympathetic but firm response very promptly, backed up by full supporting documentation including description of the stakeholder and user input. If you do this, then queries soon die down, whereas defensive, slow, inaccurate and incomplete responses lead to escalating concerns.

Case 7.1 Case study—coping with demand for ovarian cancer screening

An influential and high profile clinician in your local hospital has decided to launch a local screening service for ovarian cancer. This has been prompted by the recent death of a well-known local television presenter, mother of two young children. The clinician has written to local family doctors asking that they inform their female patients age 45 and over of the new local service, which involves an ultrasound examination and a blood test. You only hear of the plans for the screening clinic when a colleague brings the clinician's letter to your attention. The letter quotes a 1999 pilot study published in the *Lancet* (Jacobs *et al*. 1999). The proposed screening clinic is about to receive a donation of £50 000 from public fundraising following the television presenter's death.

Case 7.1 Case study—coping with demand for ovarian cancer screening *(cont.)*

What do you do?

The first task is to check on the national policy and standards for ovarian screening and for gynaecological cancer services in general.

This tells you that a systematic review of the evidence relating to ovarian cancer screening was published in the year before the pilot study report (Bell *et al.* 1998), there is a major multicentre randomized controlled trial of screening in progress (UK Collaborative Trial of Ovarian Cancer Screening website), the national recommendation is that routine screening should only take place as part of high quality research and the potential harms of screening are not insignificant. National guidance relating to the standards that must be met by gynaecological cancer services generally is not yet fully met in your local services, and a peer review visit that will assess adherence to this guidance is due in 9 months time.

The next task, equipped with this information, is to go and see the hospital clinician to find out about the plans for the screening service, and for the womens' cancer services in general. It may well be that the screening clinic is a plan that he or she has been 'bounced' into because of media interest. Once you work through with the clinician the consequences of starting to offer a screening service, then you may be able to reach agreement about more worthwhile ways in which the £50 000 donation could be used. The particular factors you would be pointing out would include:

- ◆ The national screening committee does not recommend ovarian screening except as part of high quality research.

- ◆ A major randomized controlled trial, the UK Collaborative Trial of Ovarian Cancer Screening (UKCTOCS), is in progress involving 14 centres. Until the trial is complete, there is no certainty about the benefit or harm of screening.

- ◆ The 'sorting' stage of screening involves considerable intervention, with most women having general anaesthetic to allow laparascopic inspection and usually removal of their ovaries.

Case 7.1 Case study—coping with demand for ovarian cancer screening *(cont.)*

For this reason, the protocol in the UKCTOCS is set to achieve relatively high specificity with consequently low sensitivity. A local service will be highly vulnerable to criticism when there are complications from surgery and when diagnoses arise in women who were screen negative. Without any defined quality standards, it will be impossible to defend the service from criticism.

♦ General Medical Council guidance on informed consent means that all patients offered ovarian screening must be told of the potential harm, and the uncertainty of benefit.

♦ Simple workload calculations, using the numbers of women over 45 in the population served by the hospital, will reveal that a single clinic with a one-off resource of £50 000 will rapidly become swamped with work. The surgical workload generated will lengthen the waiting times for symptomatic women. This could lead to poorer outcomes in these women, and will mean the hospital fails to meet its targets for cancer treatment waiting times. This will mean that the hospital will receive an adverse report at the forthcoming peer review visit.

♦ Discussion of the overall standards achieved by the womens' cancer treatment services is sure to reveal that some aspects of national guidance are not met and require more investment. You can point out that if the service is choosing to prioritize a non-recommended activity then they are in a weak position when arguing for more investment to meet these mandatory standards.

If these discussions go well, you may be able to agree that the new funds perhaps be used, for example, to improve the rapid access clinics, to strengthen the multidisciplinary team care, to offer better end of life support at home or to provide more family support to help partners and children going through bereavement. You will need to offer to help the clinician with communicating the reasons why this is the best use of the donated funds. If you work together

Case 7.1 Case study—coping with demand for ovarian cancer screening *(cont.)*

in dealing with the media and the fundraisers, then you will be able to resolve things effectively.

If you find that the clinician is determined to go ahead with provision of screening, then you will need to involve senior managers and board chairs and members within the hospital and within the local organization responsible for population health. You should also contact regional colleagues and those responsible for national screening programme policy, which in the UK is the national screening programmes, so that they are aware of what is happening. A quiet, firm and diplomatic approach is better than a high profile show-down. You will need to assemble information and arguments explaining the drawbacks of the screening clinic, and present this to all stakeholders. Crucial in all this is the need to emphasize the importance of high quality services for womens' cancers, and to acknowledge the commitment and dedication of the clinician who is advocating the clinic. Within that context, you can then make the case for why the stand-alone screening clinic will cause damage to women and will divert resources from what is really needed.

Problem solving in existing national programmes

We have covered how to start a screening programme (Chapter 5) and how to incorporate quality management (Chapter 6). When we run refresher days and workshops for public health practitioners, the problem that crops up the most in relation to established programmes is 'how much is the local public health practitioner actually responsible for, particularly when a local programme does not neatly match current public health administrative boundaries?'

Our answer to this is:

◆ The unique feature of the public health role locally is that you are responsible for ensuring that a high quality programme is offered to all your local resident population.

- Key requirements for this to happen are that all the parts must be in place, be resourced, be working to a good quality standard, there must be co-operation between them all and the service must be accessible to all, even to the hard to reach groups.

The trick is to strike the right balance:

- If you get too involved in the programme, you end up running things that someone else, without public health training, could handle perfectly well. The result is that your expertise and skills are not then available for tasks that really need public health skills.

- If you ignore a programme and remain completely uninvolved, then the staff do not consult you early enough when things need sorting out. It is then all too easy for relationships to break down over relatively small disagreements, for there to be no co-ordination, and no forward planning for the overall programme.

In the box below, we list some of the key national and local tasks involved in programme management.

In the UK, our approach to screening is national, and quality assurance processes are nationwide but administered at regional level, as explained in Chapter 6. It is the responsibility of these national quality assurance systems to spot shortfalls in quality, for example a laboratory that does not appear to be training its staff properly, or an invitation and reminder service that cannot demonstrate adherence to proper procedures, but the people they will write to in order to get it put right are the local director of public health and the senior managers of the organizations paying for and providing services.

Also, when a change in national policy is announced that affects more than just one service in the programme, the person who will have to take the overview, write the paper and make the case for resources is likely to be the public health practitioner.

In practice, the circumstances where local screening programmes need no public health input are virtually non-existent. All of the following would have to apply, and it is seldom that every one of these satisfactory states is in place at the same time.

Box 7.1 Local and national tasks in programme management

Screening programme management at local level

Interpreting and implementing national policy

Communicating with the local population

Identifying the eligible population

Ensuring that the service is accessible to all user groups

Co-ordinating the constituent services

Supporting and developing the staff

Reporting locally on programme performance

Ensuring that appropriate resources are available

Ensuring that information management systems are in place

Acting on recommendations from quality assurance reviews

Screening programme management at national level

Policy making

Setting and reviewing quality standards

Establishing and supporting the quality management processes

Establishing training and workforce development arrangements

Commissioning national information management systems

Factors that reduce the need for local public health input are:

- The staff running the screening are very experienced.
- The staff in the different sectors (inviting, sieving, sorting, intervening, information management and technology, training, etc.) know each other, respect each other and work well together.
- There are sufficient resources for the whole programme. A key resource is the staffing, and even where there is adequate funding for the required number of posts the actual staffing levels may be insufficient due to long-term sickness, or shortage of staff to recruit.

- The national policy is stable.
- All quality standards are being met.
- There is good quality information for participants available in different formats and languages.
- Participants find the service user-friendly and easy to access.
- Uptake levels are regarded as acceptable.
- There is agreement among all concerned about the local policy.
- The health service is not undergoing any organizational change.

At any one time it is highly likely that one or more of these factors will be posing problems, or potential problems, within your screening programme. When challenges arise, this can engender uncertainty and agitation amongst the staff involved, and this is why it is always worthwhile establishing a rapport with those delivering screening before you face such challenges. If you have taken the trouble to go and see key people, to introduce yourself, to listen to them and establish a relationship when all is fine (it does not take much time), then they are far more likely to

alert you early and work constructively with you when they are faced with a threatening external change or an internal difficulty.

The two tasks you can do that probably do most to hold programmes together and ensure that problems are solved are:

- Convene and chair a co-ordinating group for the local screening programme. This can be as infrequent as six monthly if it is a straightforward programme facing little in the way of policy changes. For complex programmes or ones that are relatively new, then three, four or even six times a year may be necessary.

- Produce an annual report that summarizes how the local programme is being delivered and managed, the activity data, the quality achieved and the forward plans. The process of producing the report requires everyone to engage and to focus on the problems that need to be addressed in the coming year. The completed report provides a means of making the programme and its achievements visible to consumer groups, and to senior staff within the organizations responsible for commissioning and providing the services.

Handling concerns about commercial sector screening

Most public health practitioners get contacted from time to time by members of the public, or by clinicians, because of issues relating to commercial sector screening. Here are some examples:

♦ The local NHS urology department puts in a business case for a new consultant surgeon purely as a result of workload arising from PSA tests done routinely on healthy men undergoing private screening. The urology department workload from transrectal biopsy, and radical surgery and radiotherapy for localized prostate cancer, has increased 10-fold in the past 5 years.

♦ A member of the public complains because she had responded to a newspaper advertisement for mobile osteoporosis screening and received confusing and inaccurate advice, including the suggestion that her husband could go for a scan and might be prescribed hormone replacement therapy.

♦ The local NHS cardiology department asks for support because several people are referred following abnormal findings on exercise electrocardiography performed as part of routine well person checks by a local private clinic. The patients are all symptom free and low risk, but the private clinic advised the patients to obtain an NHS-funded angiogram to exclude any abnormality. For people of this age and risk, with an abnormal finding on exercise testing, there is an 80 per cent chance that they do not have coronary heart disease, yet now they are worried and facing the possibility of an invasive angiography examination (see also pp. 43 and 125). None of the patients was warned of the risk of a false alarm before the test.

♦ A local radiologist contacts you because a local private hospital is offering CT scanning for osteoporosis screening. She is very concerned about the radiation dose involved and considers this practice to be dangerous and unethical.

It is not always easy to know what to do in these situations. The key issues are:

♦ Potentially harmful interventions are being offered, or promoted, to consumers without balanced information to ensure informed consent.

◆ Public sector resources are being used then to sort out the problems that private screening has uncovered, most of which are either false positives or else are conditions whose outcome would be equally good if diagnosed on the basis of symptoms.

Making a fuss locally may well be counter-productive because the present climate of public belief is so strongly in favour of any kind of screening, no matter how damaging. Public awareness concerning potential harms of poor quality and non-evidence-based screening is very much in its infancy. Very few people question the naïve belief that private screening must be saving countless lives. Even scientifically trained investigative journalists have trouble believing that public sector policy might be based on an assessment of evidence, whilst private sector policy is driven by the profit motive.

There are some signs that this may be beginning to change:

◆ In August 2004, the Consumer Association's *Which?* magazine (*Which?* 2004) reviewed five private screening clinics in England and was strongly critical of all of them. *Which?* highlighted the misleading and unbalanced information for potential participants, and the poor evidence base for many of the tests on offer.

◆ The US Food and Drug Administration has published a very clear statement on their website warning consumers about the ineffectiveness and the harms from whole-body CT screening (US Food and Drug Administration 2005).

◆ The British Medical Association in 2005 gave a clear warning that consumers should beware of *ad hoc* and unregulated screening tests, particularly those offered over the Internet (British Medical Association Board of Science 2005).

This type of pressure from expert bodies and consumer organizations exerted at a national level is important for combating misleading promotional claims concerning screening. With this national backing, then local information and publicity can also play a part.

So if you encounter misleading claims, or potentially harmful screening from private providers, or screening that leaves people without support and in need of further investigations, it is worth considering the following actions:

◆ Collect the exact details

- Contact the private provider asking for their policy, quality standards, evidence base and patient information

- Notify relevant consumer standards organizations and/or health departments for your region or country

- Inform local health service staff, including family doctors, of your concerns by using existing newsletters. This means they will be adequately briefed should any of their patients ask for advice

- If concerns are very serious and persist, then with help from a relevant press office you may decide to contact local and national media to explain your concerns.

Screening and the law

> You're a firefighter. You arrive at a burning house and hear screaming. There are ten people inside. You run in and save nine lives, but despite your best efforts, one person perishes. So, should you be cited for heroism—or indicted for homicide?
>
> Richard M. DeMay (1996)

This is how Richard DeMay in a 1996 editorial (DeMay 1996) summed up the lot of those doing screening. He was writing from a US perspective, and his article was entitled 'To err is human—to sue, American'. The American situation is not directly comparable with the rest of the world, but, despite this, concern about the legal handling of screening cases is fairly universal. This is because it stems from two factors:

- Public expectations of screening are artificially high and are inevitably shared by lawyers and judges

- There is ambiguity concerning liability for failure to prevent. At best, screening can only reduce risk, it can never eradicate it, therefore it will **always** fail to prevent some, and with some programmes most, cases. Yet the existence of a screening programme causes blame to be ascribed to the programme for any cases that do occur.

When people feel let down by screening, they frequently seek legal advice. In the majority of these cases, the lawyers for the claimant and the lawyers for the health service provider agree a financial settlement without taking the case to court. Compensation is paid without negligence being admitted or proved. The matter is settled 'out of court'. It is very expensive to defend a case through the courts, and the health service would not want to incur such an expense unless they are sure that the case will be dismissed. This can create the impression that cases have been 'won', and newspaper reports sometimes imply that this has happened, even though the cases have not been examined in court, and no case law has been established.

Screening test results such as mammography films, or cervical cytology slides, are usually sent by the claimants' lawyers to expert witnesses, who are asked to give their opinion as to whether the disease that is now known to have developed could have been detected from the screening tests. Invariably the expert witnesses conclude that an abnormality is discernible. Two crucial biases are operating here. In legal terminology they are called 'outcome' bias and 'context' bias.

- **Outcome bias.** For screening tests that involve visual perception, there is always subjective judgement involved. The witness who is asked to examine the screening test does so in full knowledge that disease has now occurred. In other words, they know the outcome. This inevitably influences their judgement of what they see. In contrast, the screener who examined the test as one of many in their routine work did not have this knowledge, because the outcome had not happened and was unknowable. Outcome bias can easily be demonstrated by giving samples to competent screeners either with or without information (true or false) telling them that disease developed subsequently (Austin 1997).

- **Context bias.** The witness examining the test can take as long as they like, hours if necessary. They can consult picture libraries and come back to examining the specimen as many times as they like. The witness is a medically qualified consultant, with 5 years medical training, at least 5 years' postgraduate training and probably many years of experience working in pathology or radiology. In contrast, the screener had to examine the test in a matter of minutes during a routine working day. The screener has been trained in the competencies required for screening, but is far less qualified than the expert witness. The screener has to strike a balance between calling too many tests positive (resulting in false alarms and overtreatment), and calling too many negative, (resulting in undetected cases). So the context in which the expert witness examines the test is entirely different from the context in which the screener examines the test.

In the UK, these crucial biases have not until recently been adequately recognized in legal proceedings.

Case 7.2 Case study—cervical screening cases in the English courts

The Kent and Canterbury cases

Problems within the cervical screening service at Kent and Canterbury Hospitals NHS Trust came to light in 1996. It transpired that the laboratory screeners were inadequately trained and supervised, and that problems had been voiced within the Trust for several years but had been ignored. More than 90 000 women had their tests re-examined, and the Trust paid more than £1 million in settlements to 47 women. Sir William Wells chaired an Inquiry (Wells 1997), following which all local NHS cervical screening programmes in England and Wales were reviewed. Strengthened nationwide quality assurance processes were put in place under the responsibility of Regional Directors of Public Health (see also Chapter 1, p. 24 and Chapter 6, p. 173).

Amongst cases contested by the Kent and Canterbury Trust were those of three women who had developed endocervical cancer following negative screening results.

The case of these three women—*Penney, Palmer and Cannon v East Kent Health Authority*—went to court and was concluded in February 1999. Judge Peppitt QC found in favour of the claimants on the grounds that the Bolam principle did not apply and that the defence did not withstand logical argument.

The Bolam test relies upon the principle that a doctor is not negligent if he acts in accordance with a practice accepted at the time as proper by a responsible body of medical opinion. The defendant's experts all testified that the screeners had acted reasonably in classifying the samples as negative. The judge concluded that because there were suspicious cells on the slides, observed by the claimant's expert witnesses, and because of the 'potentially

Case 7.2 Case study—cervical screening cases in the English courts (*cont.*)

disastrous consequences' of failing to recommend further investigation, the defendants were negligent and in breach of duty in failing to classify the appearances as at least borderline. The case did not rest on demonstration of actual harm arising from the classification of the screening tests as negative, but only on the women being denied the possibility of more conservative treatment.

This judgement ignores the very character of screening. Most particularly, it ignores the following two features:

- The nature of the screening task, involving rapid assessment of a slide containing up to 300 000 cells

- The need for a compromise between sensitivity and specificity, between medically induced harm for healthy individuals and undetected cases.

The judge relied upon the evidence of the claimants' expert witnesses who, with the benefit of hindsight and with hours to spend examining the slides, found evidence of borderline abnormality. He was judging the screening examination against the standards required of a definitive diagnostic test.

The implication of this judgment meant that a service meeting every contemporary quality standard could still potentially be judged liable if an expert witness could find abnormal cells in a previous cytology screening sample. The case went to the Court of Appeal.

On 16 November 1999, the Court of Appeal (Lord Woolf MR, May and Hale LJJ) gave judgement in the cases of *Penney, Palmer and Cannon v East Kent Health Authority*. At that stage, the three cases were the only cases on liability to have reached trial following the inquiry conducted by Sir William Wells. They attracted widespread publicity.

The Court of Appeal formulated the issues before the trial judge as 3-fold:

- What was to be seen on the individual slides

- Whether, at the relevant time, a screener exercising reasonable care could fail to see what was on the slide

Case 7.2 Case study—cervical screening cases in the English courts *(cont.)*

◆ Whether a reasonably competent screener, aware of what a screener exercising reasonable care would observe on the slide, could treat the slide as negative.

At the initial trial, the judge had accepted the evidence of the claimants' experts, Professors Krauz and Cotton, that in each of the three cases a screener exercising reasonable skill and care could not have failed to see obvious abnormalities on the slides. The Court of Appeal upheld this judgement. Lord Woolf maintained that the existence of abnormal cells on the slides was a matter of fact, whereas the claim that a competent screener under ordinary working conditions was acting reasonably in classifying the slides as negative was a matter of opinion. The cases were all adenocarcinoma cases, which are accepted as difficult to detect through screening, and the Court of Appeal expressed the view that the cases turned very much on their own facts. Despite this, the Court of Appeal decision has had a widespread impact on litigation arising out of cervical screening.

Taylor versus Barnsley Health Authority

Later the same year, a cervical screening case in the North of England was taken to court and this time the outcome was different. The case *Taylor v Barnsley Health Authority* reached court on 21 December 1999 at Sheffield County Court. As soon as the claimant's expert witness, Professor Cotton, was cross-examined, the trial judge concluded that his evidence was unconvincing and entered judgement in favour of the Health Authority. The claimant consented to judgement at the end of the evidence of her expert witness. Professor Cotton had maintained that a single abnormal cell, on a slide containing usually between 100 000 and 200 000 cells, if not seen by the screener, would mean the screener was negligent. In the language of newspaper reporters, this would be described as 'the case collapsed'.

Screening cases pose real difficulties for both claimants' and defendants' lawyers trying to evaluate the merit of each claim. Each case involves a personal tragedy for the claimant.

Case 7.2 Case study—cervical screening cases in the English courts *(cont.)*

The *Taylor* case is important because it shows that in claims where there are small numbers of abnormal, or possibly abnormal cells, the defendant is able to succeed.

Pidgeon versus Doncaster Health Authority

In another case, *Pidgeon v Doncaster Health Authority* in October 2001, issues on causation were raised in an area where there is very little case law. Although in this case breach of duty was admitted, Mrs Pidgeon's conduct in repeatedly failing to attend for screening had also been a factor. This raised important issues about the scope of the duty of care, causation and contributory negligence. The case was an important test case for cases where a claimant had refused or failed to attend for screening or subsequent tests.

The judgement, by an experienced circuit judge, rejected the submissions of the Health Authority on the scope of the duty of care and causation but found that the claimant was two-thirds responsible for her condition.

The importance of this case lies in the acceptance by the trial judge that the claimant had a responsibility to participate in the screening programme. It is now open to defendants in appropriate cases to argue that where a claimant has refused or failed to attend for screening, and the consequences of not doing so have been explained and appreciated, preferably supported by well-documented family doctor records and a family doctor witness statement, there should be a substantial reduction in the amount of damages.

It is very much in the public interest to establish a sound legal framework for screening. Staff who are meeting contemporary standards need to know that they will not fall foul of the law, and screening participants who genuinely suffer harm due to proven negligence need access to compensation. Without sound legal judgments, not only will the litigation costs associated with screening become prohibitive, but the pressures on individual screeners will make it exceedingly difficult to recruit and retain staff.

Court judgements in the USA

In Virginia USA, a court found in favour of the plaintiff when he sued his doctor for failing to perform a PSA test (Merenstein 2004). The doctor, Daniel Merenstein, on performing a routine physical examination, had discussed with the 53-year-old patient the pros and cons and the controversy surrounding PSA testing, and had documented this in the patient's records. A different doctor subsequently ordered a PSA test routinely and it transpired that the patient had a Gleason eight (the Gleason score is a measure of prognosis) incurable cancer, which probably would not have been amenable to detection or intervention at a localized stage. Nevertheless, the court judged that 'usual practice' was to perform PSA testing without prior discussion or shared decision making. Dr Merenstein's employers were found liable for US$1million.

Cases like this are extremely disturbing as they threaten the viability of efficient and effective screening programmes. It is wrong, however, to assume that litigation happening in the USA today will be happening in the rest of the world tomorrow. In the USA, because individuals are responsible for the costs of their care if they are sick, the law is used as a means of seeking finance in a way that substitutes in effect for the 'safety net' of the welfare state that many other countries are used to. For example, the differences between the situation in the USA and that in the UK are demonstrated by the way in which potential damage from silicone breast implants has been dealt with on each side of the Atlantic. It has not been an issue in the UK, yet in the USA it has brought major corporations to the brink of financial ruin. Marcia Angell describes these events in her fascinating book *Science on trial* (Angell 1990), and she analyses some of the features of American society, and its corporate, legal and health systems, that drive the commonplace pursuit of lawsuits and the astonishingly non-evidence-based judgements that are made. In Texas in 1992, for example, Pamela Johnson successfully sued Bristol-Myers Squibb for damages relating to vague complaints (sore throats, bladder infections) claimed to result from her silicone breast implants. She was awarded a record US$25 million settlement. Yet the evidence that silicone causes adverse effects other than local reactions is non-existent.

The overall conclusion is that legal aspects of screening are important. Some general messages are that:

- Local programmes need to:
  - make sure that screening meets the required quality standards
  - keep good records
  - share information with regional and national colleagues about potential incidents, important complaints or potential legal challenges.

- National and regional staff need to:
  - support local programmes in meeting quality standards
  - ensure that public information about screening gives accurate and balanced information about the limitations as well as the benefits of screening
  - ensure that the respective duties of the programme and of the person to whom screening is offered are clearly stated
  - support local programmes in dealing with potential litigation
  - secure uniform high quality legal support for national screening programmes so that appropriate cases are properly defended in court with a sharing of costs.

Handling the media

Dealing with screening in the media spotlight is particularly tricky. Every word you say has the potential to upset a viewer, listener or reader who believes their cancer could have been avoided, or their child's heart condition could have been detected before birth. Unless you come across as genuinely caring about what is best for people, and unless you make your arguments and concerns sound concrete and credible, then radio and television in particular will not be kind to your case.

Dos and don'ts of dealing with the media

Here are some general rules:

- Do find an experienced press officer (or communications officer as they tend now to be called) and get his or her help and advice.

- Do involve the regional and or national team if the issue relates to a specific programme. They can also enlist help from their press office if appropriate.

- Do warn and brief senior colleagues locally if there is going to be any adverse publicity (directors of public health, senior managers, chairs of boards) and, if family doctor practices are likely to be consulted by worried members of the public, warn them too.

- Do prepare carefully for an interview. Picture in your mind someone who represents the 'ordinary punter'—think of a typical acquaintance who you find it tricky to explain complex health issues to. If you can assemble simple facts and arguments that would make sense to this person, then you are likely to get your message across.

- Do jot down the key facts and arguments and then assemble them into a mind map. Then highlight the five or six things that are most relevant, and that are possible to put across simply. Cross out any facts and arguments that lead you into areas too complex to deal with in a short interview. Rehearse the five or six highlighted statements.

- Don't use dry academic arguments. If what you say would make sense to an intelligent 10 year old then it is probably useful, if not then choose a different line of argument. Keep things concrete not abstract, and use examples.

- Don't use the terms 'saving money' or 'a waste of money'. By all means mention the resources needed for screening (staff, equipment, training, etc.) and quote financial figures if it is about planned investment. If you are trying to explain why a certain type of screening is not being funded, then it is safer to use arguments such as 'if we were going to fund this then we would have to give up doing this, that and the other in order to afford it'. If something is ineffective, then say that it will not make any difference to the number of people who get the disease, rather than saying it is a waste of money. When people hear the word 'money' they automatically conclude that the arguments are nothing to do with benefit and harm, they are only about money.

- Don't just say 'there's no evidence'. Instead talk about what research is taking place, what other things are being done to improve prevention, prompt recognition and treatment, and explain that until there is certainty about benefit, one has to be influenced by the certain knowledge that screening will bring some harm.

- Don't try and be lighthearted about screening. There is always a danger that this will come across as flippant and uncaring, and taken out of context it can be very damaging.

Classic interview questions

In Table 7.1 we have assembled some of the classic questions that get asked in media interviews about screening, and we illustrate some of the more effective ways of coping with these questions. We have used PSA (prostate-specific antigen) testing as an example.

Table 7.1 Classic interview questions and how to handle them

Interviewer: 'I've got a huge list here of prestigious organizations all of them calling for immediate introduction of screening for prostate cancer. It's absolutely outrageous that men are being denied this important service. How on earth can you defend this position?"	
Weak answer	'Most prostate cancers are not harmful. Screening would be very expensive and we do not have enough evidence'.
Comment	This sounds a bit defensive, it sounds as though you just want to avoid the expense, and the statement about prostate cancer not being harmful runs so counter to most people's beliefs that a lot of listeners will immediately conclude that you are mad and will therefore disregard all your subsequent statements.
Stronger answer	'We have learned a great deal about screening in the last 40 years. We have learned that if you don't research the screening properly before you start, and if you don't organize a proper national programme, with training, with quality standards, and with adequate resources, then screening definitely leads to more harm than good. Important research is taking place into prostate screening, but from what we know at present it would definitely do more harm than good if we introduced a programme'.

Table 7.1 (continued) Classic interview questions and how to handle them

Comment	You are establishing yourself from the outset as someone who is happy to talk about screening, you sound interested in engaging the listeners in the issues. This is a good starting point and will enable you to build your case.

Interviewer: 'But there are countless men who testify to the value of this test. Award-winning actor Robert de Niro, Yankees manager Joe Torre, former mayor of New York Rudy Guiliani, US Senator Bob Dole, retired General Norman Schwarzkopf … the list goes on. All of them say they owe their lives to the test. You are flying in the face of all this evidence'.

Weak answer	'You cannot base a screening programme just on anecdotal evidence. They may think they have had their lives saved but they are probably wrong. We have to have RCT evidence'.
Comment	The listeners will probably just think that this sounds arrogant and narrow-minded, even though it is all accurate and legitimate. The interviewer can counter you with questions such as 'this just sounds like a delaying tactic, how many men have to die before you will act?' or 'the cervical screening programme is highly successful, and it was introduced without randomized controlled trial evidence'
Stronger answer	'Lots of men have changes in their prostates that look like cancer but are not behaving like cancer. Men die with these changes, not of them. So when these men are treated and do well, they think their life has been saved, but most of them would never have developed full-blown cancer. This happens with many types of screening. Let me give you an example—infant screening for a tumour called neuroblastoma has now been proven to make no difference whatsoever to the serious cases but leads to dangerous, sometimes even fatal, treatment in infants who would never have developed a problem. The same happens with prostate screening. We offer very invasive treatments— radical surgery or radiotherapy—to men who were never going to develop cancer. Serious side effects are common, and we have no idea how effective these treatments are at stopping anyone dying of prostate cancer. The harm is definite, the benefit is only a possibility'.
Comment	You have managed to focus again on what this is really about, which is harm and benefit. You have dealt with the popularity paradox issue (see p. 68) without falling into the trap of appearing to imply that ordinary people are being stupid.

Interviewer: 'We spend hundreds of millions of pounds every year on screening for women's cancers but you sit there and tell me that men can't have prostate screening. This is grossly unfair'.

Table 7.1 (continued) Classic interview questions and how to handle them

Weak answer	'There are doubts as to whether the money spent for women's cancer screening is money well spent. Prostate cancer screening would be very expensive indeed, and most men dying of prostate cancer are very elderly'.
Comment	Mentioning controversy about women's cancer screening will probably convince all the listeners (apart from any in public health) that you are completely unhinged. They will conclude that not only do you not care about men, you do not care about women either, and you seem to be ageist.
Stronger answer	'This is not about money. If you handed me a cheque for £500 million I would not, on current evidence, spend it on prostate screening. Until we know more about interventions that definitely stop men developing metastatic prostate cancer, and that are safe, then screening is the wrong thing to be doing'.
Comment	You are emphasizing yet again that if we really care about the good of the people's health then the argument is about whether prostate screening is worthwhile, does it definitely do more good than harm. Until this is resolved, then arguments about affordability are pointless.

Interviewer: 'Prostate screening is provided in America, France and Germany. It's an absolute disgrace that the UK is lagging behind by not providing it'.

Weak answer	'These countries spend more on their health services than we do in the UK. We have to be certain that screening is cost-effective before we introduce it'.
Comment	This suggests that the issue is more about affordability than about benefit and harm. The listener may think that you just do not want to pay for it.
Stronger answer	'There are important differences between the health services in the countries you mention, and the health service in the UK. In this country, we take the view that where screening is definitely worthwhile and affordable then it will be provided as a high quality national programme available to everybody. The situation in the USA, France and Germany is that private clinics offer all kinds of screening tests. Because they are well advertised, consumers assume that the tests must be helpful but it's not what we would recognize as a quality screening programme'.
Comment	This answer commends the national approach instead of letting people assume that we are lagging behind. It emphasizes that we have equity of access and a national grip on things.

Dealing with quality failures

If you are handling media interviews regarding a potential or known problem relating to quality within an existing national programme, then some key points to follow are:

+ Always praise the work of the staff doing the screening—their dedication, the difficult and repetitive work that they do, and the quality checks, tests and exams that they comply with.

+ If there are patients or members of the public who are worried and might be needing repeat tests for example, explain clearly what help and information is available for them, and acknowledge that you recognize their concern.

+ Stress how much the service is valued—even if a problem has come to light in one aspect, the vast majority of recipients of screening are very appreciative of the service.

+ Emphasize that it is because of efficient systems for regularly monitoring quality that a problem has been immediately spotted, and hence is in the news. Explain that the problem has been recognized, investigated and is being put right.

+ Keep things in context for the public; emphasize the other aspects of primary prevention for the disease and the importance of consulting early over any possible symptoms. Explain that screening is only one part of the overall system of care for the disease in question.

+ Distinguish between problems that are due to avoidable quality failure, versus problems that are inherent limitations and are unavoidable. Explain that these limitations exist in even the highest quality programmes the world over, i.e. cases that are undetectable, cases that have a poor outcome despite being picked up on screening, false alarms and overtreatment for disease that would not progress.

Summary points

Provision of inappropriate screening not backed by sound evidence is bad for population health due to direct harm, diversion of resources away from valuable health service provision, and lost opportunities for well conducted randomized controlled trials.

Key steps in controlling inappropriate screening are: understanding and acknowledging the reasons for its growth, communicating clear information about why it is not in the interests of public health and introducing specific controls to ensure that policy is adhered to.

Within established national screening programmes, the public health responsibility locally is to ensure that a high quality programme is in place and is offered to all of the local resident population.

Three actions that help achieve this local public health role are: establishing a relationship with lead individuals for each component of the local programme, convening and chairing a co-ordinating group, and producing annual reports on the programme that include forward plans.

The public health input needed for a local programme varies. It is least when the staff in the programme are experienced and work well together across different organizations, resources are sufficient, policy is stable, quality standards are met and the health service is not undergoing structural reorganization.

Public health concerns about private sector screening include worries that consumers are given inadequate or even misleading information, are offered tests likely to do more harm than good and are left with positive findings and no further investigations, interventions or support.

It may be worthwhile to raise concerns about inappropriate or poor quality private sector screening with the providers themselves, with relevant regional and national colleagues, with consumer protection authorities and possibly with the media.

In legal cases concerning screening, out of court settlements to claimants are common even where the screening service has met

Summary points *(cont.)*

all the required quality standards. This is because no provider wants the costs of fighting a case in court. Better legal support is needed for national screening programmes in order that appropriate cases can be expertly defended with sharing of costs.

Important screening case law was established in a 1999 cervical screening case *Taylor v Barnsley Health Authority*. This case shows that it is possible to expose the unreasonableness of expert testimony which ignores context bias and outcome bias.

There are some important dos and don'ts for handling media interviews relating to screening. Get help from an experienced press officer, prepare well, always talk in terms of benefit and harm, never be flippant, do not talk about saving money but explain the trade-offs, talk positively about wanting to improve services and prevention, and use simple explanations rather than dry academic arguments.

When interviewed about a service quality problem, always praise the staff, emphasize the difficult nature of the work and mention the quality checks and proficiency tests. Explain that the problem has come to light because of the rigorous quality management systems, and explain what is being done to put things right.

Test yourself

Question one

You are the public health lead for children's health working in an English city. You discover that several of your local family doctors are offering routine screening for anaemia for all infants registered with their practices. This began as a small research study aimed at finding out the prevalence of iron deficiency anaemia amongst infants in a multicultural area. The practices found a higher than expected prevalence. They are continuing to do tests routinely and have now submitted a business case to your department seeking funding to continue the routine screening tests for anaemia for all infants in their practices.

To answer questions one and two, look on the world wide web to find out what the policy recommendations and evidence are in relation to iron deficiency screening in infants. On the basis of what you find, decide what action you would take.

Question two

The local radio station phones up asking for an interview about the infant screening service for anaemia. One of the family doctors will be in the studio. You have the choice of declining to be interviewed, joining in on a phone line or going and participating in the studio. What would you do, and, if you do agree to be interviewed, what are the main 'soundbites' you will want to get across?

Question three

You are the public health lead for your local cervical screening programme. Four years ago the local nursing director with responsibility for staff training for screening sample takers established a successful 2-day training course for sample takers, and a half-day refresher course. These are run regularly at the training centre, are well attended, well evaluated and meet the national specification for the required content of sample taker training. The nursing director contacts you because the funding for running the courses is going to be withdrawn. This is because the training confederation that allocated the funding is going to be abolished as part of a restructuring. What do you do?

Question four

You receive through the post at home a leaflet advertising a local health screening clinic. The screening that they offer includes hair analysis, live blood analysis and the use of an electrodiagnostic device that measures polarization values within the skin. You look these techniques up on the web and discover that all are strongly criticized and some have been the subject of legal prosecutions against practitioners using them. You do not have a lot of time on your hands. What would you do?

Chapter 8

Making screening policy

All screening debates are debates between snails
and evangelists

Sackett and Holland (1975)

The aim of this chapter

After reading this chapter, you will have an appreciation of how evidence can be used for policy making. You will also understand how resources, values and beliefs all influence screening policy, and you will have insight into some of the ethical dilemmas involved. You will recognize the need for following robust and explicit processes when making screening policy, and that this is best done at national level.

Making policy about health service provision is never easy, and screening is no exception. Whenever screening policy decisions are faced, problems arise because:

- There may be a lack of appreciation of the biases that can affect screening data, and of the full range of outcomes that need to be considered. This can mean that scrutiny and interpretation of evidence may not happen as rigorously as they should. There have been examples where decisions about screening policy have used very limited evidence, invalid evidence, confusing and misleading formats for the evidence, and evidence that is slanted one way or another. The way that evidence is presented has been shown to have a profound influence on decisions.

- Culturally determined beliefs and values in society have a strong influence on decision makers and consumers. Belief that all screening must automatically be a good thing is very strong. There is a feeling that even when the evidence is against screening, it must still be some use because at least you are 'doing something'. Society's values enter the debate when it comes to choosing whether every individual has a right to everything, whether fairness is important and whether value for money should be allowed to have an influence.

- Commercial factors and other interests, such as the status of an individual or institution and the ability to attract research grants, may lie behind much of the pressure for screening, but these motives are seldom apparent to decision makers or to the public, who tend to assume that lobbyists are motivated only by an interest in the population's health. Commercial influences are often invisible. They may be achieved by funding of patient support groups to put pressure on decision makers, by third party techniques for lobbying governments, by planting stories in the media and by enlisting celebrity endorsement.

- Single issue lobbying can lead to disproportionate action. Policy decisions that bring most benefit across the whole population, or for all people affected by a particular disease, are difficult to achieve when a single issue is given high profile and no context.

- Ethical conflicts feature strongly when weighing up good, harm and affordability, and when deciding how to promote screening and inform the public. Is it acceptable, for example, to cause death in a healthy person in order to benefit others? Is it acceptable to gloss over the risks if this could encourage the hard-to-reach groups to attend? There is no single set of ethical principles to guide judgements about screening policy. Principles of individual rights, justice and greatest good for the greatest number can assist, but often all they do is illustrate that given any difficult decision there could be several answers.

- Conflict exists between what people need (the capacity to experience measurable benefit in health), what people demand and what people want. If you ask pressure groups arguing for prostate screening why it is that they want it, they are more likely to say 'because they have it in the USA', than to say 'because we are certain it will do more good than harm'. There are many reasons why members of the public, healthcare providers and politicians 'want' screening, and often these are not related to any direct benefit from screening itself. For example, screening may be seen as the best way of raising the profile of a disease, of attracting investment or of convincing the voting public that the government cares about health.

♦ Resources are never sufficient for all the healthcare activity that providers want to deliver and that people want to receive, so difficult choices are unavoidable.

Who makes policy decisions about screening?

For screening, decisions about policy are generally made for a whole population at either national or regional level. True-life policy making seldom follows the neat stepwise sequence that we might theoretically expect. In addition, there is considerable variation internationally in the way that screening is decided upon, provided, regulated and quality assured.

In the UK, there is a national screening committee advising the four health departments (for Wales, Scotland, Northern Ireland and England) on national policy decisions for screening in the National Health Service. If the policy is to provide quality-assured screening then this is delivered as a nationally monitored programme. Most of the provision is by public sector organizations, although some components of the services may be contracted from the independent sector.

Policy decisions in some countries relate more to the question of what services are or are not reimbursed from public funds, with provision being delivered and regulated by a mix of public and private providers. This is the situation in Australia and Canada.

Sometimes policy is concerned only with whether a given activity is recommended. Such recommendations may be national, or local. It is then up to each consumer to decide if they can afford a health insurance policy that includes the screening activity. This is the situation in the USA.

What kind of decisions have to be made?

The two main types of screening policy decision are:

♦ **Starting screening, or stopping screening from starting:** should there or should there not be a screening programme for a given health problem? If there should be a screening programme, then what 'recipe' should be used; what test, what frequency, what eligible population, what sorting process, what intervention, what thresholds? Should a demonstration or pilot site be launched to test out the implementation? If there should not be a screening programme, then can and should haphazard provision of screening be actively discouraged or even stopped from starting (see Chapter 7, p. 181). If evidence is lacking, then should research be commissioned?

◆ **Changing existing screening:** for an existing screening programme, should the recipe be changed, for example to alter the frequency, the test, the sorting process, the intervention or the eligible population?

Additional questions that policy makers are faced with include:

◆ What approach should be taken to providing information for potential participants? For example, should information be designed solely to encourage participation, or should there be an emphasis on balanced information and individual choice even at the expense of uptake? What information should be actively given, and what information should be available on request?

◆ How much central control should there be to ensure that the screening is delivered as a public health programme to the whole population?

How screening policy decisions are made

There are four main factors:

◆ Evidence
◆ Resources
◆ Values
◆ Beliefs.

Commercial influences play a part and these operate by influencing all four of the factors listed above.

Evidence and resources

If life were simple, then all you need to do to make screening policy is:

◆ look at the evidence concerning benefit, harm and value for money, and

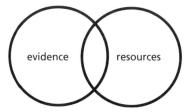

Fig. 8.1 Factors in policy making: evidence and resources.

- take a decision on the basis of how much resource you have and what other needs you have to meet (Fig. 8.1).

The UK National Screening Committee has drawn up and published explicit criteria (National Screening Committee 2003) aimed at formalizing this logical approach.

But of course, life is not that simple. The fundamental difficulties are:

- Weighing up and judging evidence relating to the magnitude of benefit, magnitude of harm and value for money compared with other options is highly complex and subjective. Simple 'yes/no' answers cannot easily be determined for each of the criteria, and almost no existing programme has unqualified 'yes' answers for every one.

- The values and beliefs held by society have a profound influence on decision making at every level within the health service.

- Policy decisions are inevitably influenced, to a greater or lesser extent, by commercial factors.

We will come to the influence of values, beliefs, and commercial factors later in the chapter. First we need to look at some of the challenges faced in assessing evidence for policy making. Chapter 4 dealt with the problem of what constitutes valid evidence about screening. What we are concerned with now is the way that evidence is presented. By evidence we mean information about the benefit and harms, and about the resources needed to deliver the screening programme.

For policy making it is not sufficient to know only what level of resources will be needed for the screening programme, you also need to know the amount of resources you have available to use for improving health. This includes factors such as whether you have a trained workforce capable of delivering screening, whether you have sufficient finance to invest to achieve a high quality programme, and what other service improvements are competing for the same funding. This type of economic assessment has to be made whenever plans and priorities are being drawn up in the health service. Choices, or prioritization, or rationing decisions are made all the time in healthcare, and there is nothing special about the decisions made in relation to screening.

There are advantages to taking screening decisions centrally:

♦ If the decision is that screening will be provided, then a national approach makes it easier to achieve an equitable and high quality service.

♦ If the decision is that screening will not be provided, then a national decision, taken on the basis of high quality evidence and through a robust process, is more likely to be influential in protecting the public from the harms of haphazard growth of unvalidated screening. Requiring the decision to be made a hundred times over, by each small local institution, brings many problems. Small organizations seldom have the resources to document meticulously all the detail of evidence and process for decision making in a way that can withstand skilful legal challenge from 'access advocates' backed up by resources from those who stand to gain commercially (Mayer 2005; Moynihan and Cassels 2005). For example, in the UK, when public sector decision making is challenged in the courts through Judicial Review, the lawyers are not judging whether a decision is the right one for improving public health. They are scrutinizing the process, often in a way that is divorced from the real life context of small healthcare organizations dealing day to day with multiple complex challenges.

♦ A national process also stands a better chance of guiding appropriate decisions about necessary research.

Using evidence for policy making

Policy makers need valid evidence, presented clearly and fairly. Important considerations are:

♦ Ease of understanding
♦ Framing effects

- Balanced presentation
- Asking the right questions about costs
- Asking programme questions, not single issue questions.

Making evidence understandable

Gerd Gigerenzer is a psychologist who has researched and written extensively about the way people understand and interpret risk, uncertainty and probability. His conclusion is that most of us find statistical presentations highly confusing, even though we can readily understand the same information when it is shown in a way that matches how most of us think.

This illustrates the difference it makes, even for highly qualified people, if information is presented in the way we experience it in real life. Gigerenzer defines natural frequencies as numbers that correspond to the way humans experienced information before the invention of probability theory. This means using 'raw' numbers of people and numbers of events, preferably with the kind of numbers it is easy

---

Case 8.1 Case study—physicians' understanding of positive screening results

Gigerenzer and his colleague Ulrich Hoffrage carried out an experiment with 48 German physicians (Gigerenzer 2002). They asked the physicians about the chance of breast cancer in a woman with a positive mammogram, and they gave them the information needed to work this out. Half the physicians were given the information as natural frequencies, and half were given it as probabilities.

Natural frequencies

For a group of women participating in mammography screening, eight out of every 1000 women have breast cancer. Of these eight women with breast cancer, seven will have a positive mammogram. Of the remaining 992 women who do not have breast cancer, 70 will still have a positive mammogram.

Question: for a woman with a positive mammogram, what is the chance that she has breast cancer?

Case 8.1 Case study—physicians' understanding of positive screening results *(cont.)*

Probabilities

Probability of breast cancer = 0.008

Probability of positive result if have breast cancer = 0.875

Probability of positive if no breast cancer = 0.07

Question: for a woman with a positive mammogram, what is the chance that she has breast cancer?

The correct answer to the question—what is the chance of breast cancer in a woman with a positive mammogram—is that there are seven breast cancers out of 77 positive mammographies, which works out as one in 11, or a 9 per cent chance (7/77 × 100).

In the group given natural frequencies, 11 physicians out of the 24 gave the correct answer, and only five were wildly out, with answers above 50 per cent. One might have hoped that all would have got it right, but therein lies much of the mistaken beliefs about screening that have bedevilled the past 150 years.

Not surprisingly, Gigerenzer found that in the group given probabilities, two of the 24 physicians gave a correct answer and 16 gave wildly incorrect answers of over 50 per cent. To a statistician, the problem is solvable from the probabilities with a formula. Another method is to use the probabilities to work out the numbers amongst 1000 tested women and then solve it from these numbers. For most people though, the probability information is just unintelligible. Yet papers and reports concerning screening seldom present statistics as clear natural frequencies and, according to Gigerenzer, most medical textbooks explain information using the confusing probabilities format that he used in his study.

---

to imagine (not millions, and not decimals), and laid out in the same way that the events happen in true life. In Gigerenzer's work, he cites many more experiments and examples that confirm this phenomenon. Policy makers are no exception, and when they are looking at evidence from research they need to be able to understand what this evidence actually means in practice.

Framing

Framing is the jargon term for another phenomenon to do with the presentation of information. It relates to the fact that the same data, presented or framed in different ways, will elicit different responses and conclusions even in the same person. This has been recognized by psychologists for years. Advertisers and salespeople use this phenomenon all the time to present data in ways most likely to impress.

There are several ways in which research evidence about the magnitude of benefit, or harm, can be presented. Commonly used methods are:

◆ Relative risk reduction—to explain what this is, imagine there are six deaths in a thousand patients without treatment, and four deaths in a thousand with treatment. The relative risk reduction is the difference between six and four expressed as a percentage of six, or 2/6 × 100 = 33 per cent. In other words, deaths are cut by one-third.

◆ Absolute risk reduction—using the same example, the absolute risk reduction is the real reduction in risk for an individual, which in this case is two less chances in a thousand. As a percentage this is 0.2 per cent, as a probability it is 0.002. An individual's chance of dying is cut by one-fifth of 1 per-cent, or by one in 500.

◆ Percentage of event-free patients—this statistic gives you the percentage of patients, with and without the intervention, who do not experience the bad outcome that the study measured. So with the same example it is 994 out of a thousand versus 996 who have not died. An individual's chance of staying alive is 99.4 per cent without treatment versus 99.6 per cent with treatment.

◆ Number needed to treat—this is the number of people who have to undergo the treatment in order for one to benefit. In our example, for a thousand people who have treatment, there are two less deaths. So 500 need treatment for one person to benefit.

Case study 8.2 (see p. 224) shows that policy makers are influenced by the framing effect. Large relative risk reductions 'heart attacks cut by 50 per cent' can sound impressive. If they relate to events that have a very low absolute risk, then most people express considerable surprise when they see the contrast between relative risk reduction versus absolute reduction and numbers needed to treat (Moynihan and Cassels 2005).

Case 8.2 Case study—the effect of framing

In 1994 Tom Fahey and his colleagues conducted a study to see whether the way that evidence was framed had an effect on health policy decision makers (Fahey *et al.* 1995). Evidence from a randomized trial on breast cancer screening, and from a systematic review on cardiac rehabilitation, was presented in four different ways and sent to all 182 Board Members from Health Authorities across the Oxford region. The information was in the form of a questionnaire containing a series of statements, each using a different method of presentation. Against each statement of benefit, respondents were asked how strongly they would support the funding of the intervention.

The data sent to the health authority members are summarized below, although the respondents did not see them in this summary form. All the data relate to risk of death, from breast cancer (mammography example) or from heart attack (cardiac rehabilitation example).

Information presentation	Mammography	Cardiac rehabilitation
Relative risk reduction	34%	20%
Absolute risk reduction	0.06%	3%
Percentage of event-free patients	99.82 versus 99.8%	84 versus 87%
Number needed to treat (NNT)	1592	31

Questionnaires were completed by 140 of the study participants, and the results showed that willingness to fund either programme was influenced significantly by the way in which the results were presented. People were more likely to think that funding for either activity was a good idea when they were shown the relative risk reduction. Only three of the respondents (all lay members and claiming no training in epidemiology) said that the four sets of data could be summarizing the same results.

Balance

The way information is interpreted and judged also depends on the formats and techniques used for portraying positive and negative aspects. Advertisers have always used these techniques, with the drawbacks of products mentioned last, and only in small print. Television and film documentary makers employ numerous balance techniques, such as sinister music and harsh lighting to make certain information sound negative, and uplifting music, soft lighting and sympathetic portrayal of the advocate when they want a positive slant. In courts of law there are strict rules about the timing, sequence and method for taking evidence from prosecution and defence, all of which is aimed at achieving balance.

Information about screening that is slanted towards the positive aspects is something we are used to. The example in Table 8.1 illustrates this. We have taken three statements that used to be in the UK national leaflets about cervical screening, and applied the equivalent presentation technique to a negative aspect of screening. Negatively slanted information is definitely not something we would advocate; we use it simply to illustrate how we have come to accept unbalanced information provided it is slanted in favour of screening. The current version of the national leaflet (NHS Cancer Screening Programmes 2006) is now more balanced, and explains that screening prevents most but not all cancers of the cervix, that there are limitations to screening and that one downside is that many women experience abnormal results yet the majority of these are due to cell changes that would never cause a health problem.

Another way in which lack of balance creeps in relates to confidence intervals. Often the potential benefits of screening are stated based on the upper confidence limit of the mortality reduction found in experimental trials. For example, the Nottingham randomized trial of bowel screening (Hardcastle *et al.* 1996) found a mortality reduction of 15 per cent, with 95 per cent confidence limits of 2–26 per cent. What this means is that with a study this size, and a result of 15 per cent, then you can be 95 per cent certain that the true reduction is somewhere between 2 and 26 per cent. The Nottingham results led to statements that 'bowel screening could cut deaths by as much as 30 per cent', but not to statements that 'the impact of bowel screening could be as low as a two per cent reduction in deaths'. Professor Les Irwig, who heads up

Table 8.1 Illustration of unbalanced information

Technique	Example that used to appear in national leaflet	Example of application to a negative effect
Using a national statistic to give an impressively big number, rather than using frequency for an individual	Cervical cancer kills 2000 women each year in England and Wales	Screening causes 80 000 women to have unnecessary treatment each year in England and Wales
Dismissing a risk as unimportant because it has a low probability [Note: the chance of staying disease free after treatment for screen-detected cervical intraepithelial neoplasia is around 98 per cent (Soutter *et al.* 1997), the lifetime chance of not dying of cervical cancer without screening is around 98 per cent (Quinn *et al.* 2000)].	Treatment of screen-detected disease is virtually 100 per cent effective	It is virtually 100 per cent certain that you will not die of cervical cancer, even if you do not go for screening
Using an imprecise claim, open to misinterpretation (Note: most people interpret statements about prevention as meaning a guarantee, rather than just a reduction in risk)	Screening prevents cancer	Screening damages health

the Screening and Test Evaluation Unit at the University of Sydney's School of Public Health, has quite rightly pointed out that whenever modelling is used to estimate benefit, harm and cost for screening programmes, the model should be run using both the lower confidence limit and the upper confidence limit to give a range of predictions.

So, information for policy making should be presented in a balanced way. The same applies to information that individuals receive to help them decide whether or not to participate in screening.

In order for information to be balanced, you need to apply exactly equivalent techniques to portraying the negative and the positive. This covers everything from font size, order of presentation, tone of voice and addition of emotive adjectives. Assessment tools are being developed to help with objective assessment of balance (Elwyn *et al.* 2006).

Asking the right questions about costs

We talked in Chapter 4 about the need to assemble direct evidence concerning the resources needed to deliver high quality screening. Many policy decisions in screening depend on a proper understanding of the resources that will be required. Two important points are:

- The full costs of providing screening programmes are usually underestimated at the planning stages.

- The law of diminishing returns is very important in screening. As you add more tests, more investigations and greater frequency, you achieve smaller and smaller gains relative to the extra investment and the extra harm. To really understand value for money, you must look at the *extra* cost, benefit and harm achieved by any change. It is not enough to just look at the total effects. The technical term for this is marginal analysis. We give an example in the case study below on cervical screening frequency.

Whenever you are presented with costs for a new programme, it is worth checking these against the programme diagram on p. 131 to see whether everything has been included in the costings. The England and Wales breast screening programme, for example, was planned on the basis of a report from a committee chaired by Sir Patrick Forrest (Forrest 1986). This document included full costings for the programme. Looking back at the report after nearly 20 years, it seems extraordinary that the costs of the information technology systems for the programme, and the management costs of the service were judged to be nil, and the cost of additional pathology services was estimated solely as 12 consultant staff for the entire UK.

Whenever you are presented with information about more intense or less intense screening, you must make sure that the separate cost of the extra intensity is clear, together with the separate benefit that the extra intensity brings. The following case study shows why this is important.

Case 8.3 Case study—cervical screening frequency

Screening to prevent cancer of the cervix is routine in many countries. In most European and Scandinavian countries, it is five yearly or three yearly, whereas for women in the USA and in countries such as Germany, cervical screening used to be recommended and performed annually or even six monthly. This wide variation in frequency is not matched by any discernible difference in the impact of the different national programmes (Levi *et al.* 2000; Linos and Riza 2000; van Ballegooijen *et al.* 2000). In terms of effectiveness, the difference between five, three, two yearly or annual screening is too small to measure directly, and we therefore have to rely on case–control estimates (IARC Working Group 1986). Economic difference between the different frequencies is substantial, and has been carefully analysed and discussed by David M Eddy, a prominent champion of evidence-based health policy in the USA (Eddy 1990), and by Louise Russell, Professor of Economics at Rutgers University (Russell 1994).

First let us consider what happens to the benefit and the harm as the frequency of screening increases. The numbers shown in Table 8.2 are taken from David Eddy's work. They set out the extra benefit with each increase in frequency together with the extra harm in terms of false alarms. If screening is annual, then every woman will suffer a false positive at some stage during her screening history.

Next, we need to look at the resources needed for the different frequencies, and relate this to the estimates for the number of deaths avoided. If you do this by looking at average cost per year of life saved, this hides some important information. It is only by looking at the extra gain for each extra cost that you can see the actual effect of providing more frequent screening compared with less frequent screening. Table 8.3 shows this, with average cost in the centre column, and marginal or extra cost in the right hand column.

If you just look at the average costs, then you might conclude that annual screening is reasonable value for money, since interventions that cost US$30 000 per life year are not unheard of. However, for sound policy making, you must calculate the extra cost of achieving an extra year of life with each successive reduction in the screening interval and you must take account of the

Case 8.3 Case study—cervical screening frequency *(cont.)*

Table 8.2 Extra benefit and extra false alarms with increasing cervical screening frequency

Years between tests	Percentage reduction in cancer incidence	Percentage of women with false-positive smear tests in their lifetime
10	64.1	15
5	83.6	30
3	90.8	50
2	92.5	75
1	93.5	100

extra harm. When this is done, it shows that the extra gain from two yearly over three yearly comes at an estimated US$263 000 per life year, and causes an extra 25 per cent of women to suffer a false alarm. The extra gain from annual over two yearly comes at US$1 100 000 per life year and means that all women suffer a false alarm. You will achieve far greater health improvement by sticking with five yearly or three yearly screening and using your extra resource for other, more beneficial activities.

Of course most of what is written about cervical screening frequency just talks about what is 'best', or even what is a 'safe' policy. This assumes a very narrow view of 'best' and of 'safe' since it ignores all other possible resource needs, ignores screening-related harm and implies quite wrongly that if you spend enough on screening it will bring complete protection.

Table 8.3 Extra costs (in US dollars) per life year gained with increasing cervical screening frequency

Years between tests	Average cost per life year saved	Marginal cost per life year saved compared with frequency in the row above
4	US$10 000	
3	US$13 000	US$185 000
2	US$19 000	US$263 000
1	US$30 600	US$1 100 000

Asking programme questions, not single issue questions

It is the job of health policy makers to take account of all health needs. It is the role of single issue pressure groups, and of equipment or drug manufacturers anxious to corner the market, to persuade policy makers to ignore other health needs and think only of one issue. If information for policy making is to serve the health needs of the public to best effect, then it must enable policy makers to keep a sense of perspective and context. Doing this requires policy questions that are concerned with whole programmes of care, not just with single issues.

Case 8.4 Case study—single issue and programme questions in bowel cancer screening

Imagine you are helping make policy about screening for bowel cancer, and you are doing this for several different countries all with widely varying economic circumstances and different levels of provision within their healthcare services. Each country has the same size of population, and the resources needed for the screening programme will be the equivalent of a £50 million annual running cost in each country.

The single issue question is:

- Would bowel screening do more benefit than harm to the population?

Evidence from randomized controlled trials (Towler *et al.* 2000) shows a modest reduction in deaths from bowel cancer, and some harmful effects, but, provided that a high quality service can be delivered, then the answer to this question will be yes. The onus is then on the policy makers, or the healthcare funders, or the consumers of healthcare, to find a way of affording bowel screening.

If instead you turn the issue into a programme question, you would be asking:

- Would bowel screening be more beneficial to the population than any current healthcare activity that could be stopped (either within bowel cancer services, or across all healthcare) to release the necessary £50 million?

> **Case 8.4 Case study—single issue and programme questions in bowel cancer screening** *(cont.)*
>
> Or alternatively you might be asking:
>
> ◆ If we had an extra £50 million per year to spend (either on bowel cancer services, or on any healthcare) would bowel screening be the most beneficial thing we could do with this investment?
>
> Programme questions are more likely to result in policies that do the best for public health. In one country, the greatest benefit might come from investment in surgical services, or facilities for delivering standard chemotherapy and radiotherapy. Another country might have no community staff trained in pain control, so this investment could be the highest priority. Some countries may have comprehensive services for diagnosis treatment and care, high levels of public awareness and high consumption of fresh fruit and vegetables. In this situation, screening may well be the best investment for any new resource.

That completes our list of things to remember when using evidence for policy making, so now we need to turn to the factors aside from evidence and resources, that influence screening policy.

The importance of values

In screening, even more than in other health issues, values are a hugely influential factor. A good illustration of this is provided by the events that took place when the USA National Institutes of Health attempted to take a rationalist's view on breast screening. Harvard Professor Suzanne Fletcher, who chaired a 1993 National Cancer Institute Workshop on breast cancer, recounted the events in a *New England Journal of Medicine* editorial (Fletcher 1997).

In Fletcher's article, she likens these experiences to a scene from Lewis Carroll's book, *Alice's Adventures in Wonderland*. Like Alice, the scientists on the consensus panel had encountered problems applying evidence-based logic in an illogical world. The author of Alice, an Oxford University mathematician with a fascination for logic and illogicality, would no doubt have appreciated the mammography story.

Case 8.5 Case study—the mammography wars

The setting for this story is the USA National Cancer Institute, one of the departments of the National Institutes of Health (NIH). This world-renowned centre for medical research sprawls over the rolling hills of Bethesda, Maryland, and even has its own bus service and underground station. In 1996, the NIH organized a Consensus Conference on the issue of breast screening for women aged 40–49. A panel comprising experts and consumers examined all the relevant evidence. Their deliberations revealed considerable uncertainty as to whether any women benefit, at best less than one life might be saved if a 1000 women are screened for 10 years. The downside is that at least 250 of those 1000 women will have a positive mammogram and no benefit, and some will have cancer surgery for a tumour that is inconsequential and would never have caused a problem in the woman's lifetime. The Consensus Panel's report therefore stated that there were insufficient data to warrant recommending mammography for all women in their forties (NIH Consensus Development Panel January 1997). The Panel had approved this by a vote of 10 to 2:

> At the present time available data do not warrant a single recommendation for mammography for all women in their forties. Each woman should decide for herself whether to undergo mammography (National Institutes of Health, January 1997).

The response was dramatic.

- ◆ At the news conference announcing the report, the Panel was accused of condemning American women to death.
- ◆ The *New York Times* called the report fraudulent.
- ◆ A national television programme opened its nightly news with an apology to American women for the report.
- ◆ The Panel's chairman was summoned to the Senate Sub-Committee on Labour, Health and Human Services.
- ◆ A Senator expressed her view that the evidence favoured screening and that the Panel statement contained factual errors.

Case 8.5 Case study—the mammography wars *(cont.)*

◆ The Senate voted 98 to zero in favour of a resolution supporting mammography.

◆ Dr Richard Klausner, a molecular biologist and the head of NIH, said he was shocked by the report and asked the National Institutes of Health's Advisory Board to look at the evidence again.

The NIH Advisory Board did as they were told. They revised the recommendation from the consensus panel in a way that met with the Senate's satisfaction. The revised recommendation, issued on 27 March 1997, said that women in their forties should get a screening mammogram (NIH National Cancer Advisory Board press release March 1997). This had been approved by a vote of 17 to 1, with the only vote against being cast by an epidemiologist who had herself been diagnosed with breast cancer, not by screening, under the age of 50.

The revised recommendation was:

> Women in their forties who are at average risk should get a screening mammogram every one to two years (National Cancer Advisory Board, March 1997).

Box 8.1 The jury in Alice in Wonderland

'Let the Jury consider their verdict', the King said for about the twentieth time that day.

'No, no', said the Queen, 'sentence first—verdict afterwards'.

'Stuff and nonsense', said Alice loudly, 'the idea of having the sentence first'.

'Hold your tongue', said the Queen turning purple.

'I won't', said Alice.

'Off with her head!' the Queen shouted at the top of her voice.

Lewis Carroll: *Alice's Adventures in Wonderland*

The consensus panel looked at evidence and resources. They concluded that mammography screening for women age 40–49 does more harm than good and the resources required would do more for the public's health if used on something else. This is the evidence. What the politicians and the press, representing the public, brought to the debate were values (Fig. 8.2), and this is what the eventual decision was based on.

The values that were paramount were that if there was any potential for health improvement for an individual, then that potential should be realized, and it should be realized no matter how many resources would be needed and no matter if some women are harmed. It may be legitimate to ask whether the acquisition of these values within American society could have been influenced by the industry that depends for its commercial success on these demands. However, irrespective of how they got there, the values of society play as important a role as evidence where screening policy is concerned.

America is a highly developed country with an individualistic ethos. There is always another medical opinion to be had, and any treatment option can be pursued no matter how remote the prospects of success, just so long as you can afford it. The American medical profession has been criticized for humouring demand for their own financial ends, but that is perhaps an overcynical view of professionals who have seen themselves as pioneers in the best American tradition, members of a can-do society keen to tackle disease with all the powers at their disposal, no matter the odds stacked against the patient or the clinician.

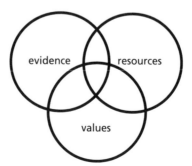

Fig. 8.2 Factors in policy making: evidence, resources and values.

Many other societies, where matters of public health are concerned, take a more collectivist approach. In these societies, it is explicitly or implicitly acknowledged that the rights of the individual to have any treatment that might be beneficial to them has to be balanced against the needs of everyone else who might need a share of the healthcare resource. The mechanisms for enacting these collectivist principles are of course under continual attack from a pharmaceutical and equipment industry using ever more inventive means to bypass traditional processes for assessment and planned introduction of new technologies.

To the Americans, collectivist societies deny their citizens the right to breast screening under the age of 50 for financial reasons or, at best, for paternalistic reasons to protect the majority from harm. To other societies, it appears that the Americans have made a recommendation about screening that will do more harm than good and that will divert much needed resources away from more beneficial activities.

It is interesting to contrast the mammography wars case study with the infant neuroblastoma screening case study in Chapter 4 (see p. 89). An American Cancer Society consensus workshop in 1991 in Chicago on neuroblastoma screening for infants recommended no screening but more research, and this was accepted (Murphy *et al.* 1991). One major difference was that at the time of the Chicago consensus workshop, neuroblastoma screening was not widespread practice in the USA, whereas mammography under 50 was already usual practice at the time of the NIH debacle. The NIH recommendation was therefore seen as denying a previously accepted practice and, as we explained in Chapter 7 (see p. 181), it can be difficult to stop screening starting, but it is even more difficult to stop it once it has started. The action of the Japanese health ministry, whereby a planned halt of their nationwide infant neuroblastoma screening programme took place once the results of the two randomized controlled trials were published (Tsubono and Hisamichi 2004), therefore has to be seen as exemplary.

The importance of beliefs

Beliefs are also important, and to examine this we will use the example of prostate screening in the UK.

Case 8.6 Case study—prostate cancer risk management

In 1996, the UK national screening committee was faced with the question of whether to recommend introduction of a national prostate screening programme.

The committee commissioned two independent systematic reviews of the evidence relating to prostate screening.

These reviews were completed in 1997 and each of them concluded that the available worldwide evidence gave no suggestion that screening for prostate cancer would do more good than harm (Chamberlain *et al.* 1997; Selley *et al.* 1997).

The appropriate policy, based on evidence and resources, would be for the National Health Service to do no prostate screening tests unless and until there was evidence to support introduction of a quality-assured national programme. However, public belief in screening was very strong, several prominent figures in British life, including Lord Steele a former cabinet minister, felt they owed their lives to the prostate-specific antigen (PSA) test, and both the *Times* and the *Daily Mail* newspapers (Cross 2002) had been actively campaigning for a screening programme. The public perception was that the government's failure to implement any screening programmes for men showed that they only cared about women dying of cancer, and government ministers shared the public's firm belief that cancer screening must be a good thing. Once ministers became aware that a no screening decision was proposed, this began to threaten the continued existence of a national framework for overseeing screening. The result was a compromise. At the press conference in February 1998, the national screening committee announced that:

+ A national screening programme for prostate cancer would not be introduced at that time, but the evidence would be kept under review.

+ Men should not routinely be offered testing within the NHS.

+ If an individual man requested a PSA test, and had been fully counselled about the possibility of harm and the uncertainty of benefit, then the NHS would provide him with a test.

> **Case 8.6 Case study—prostate cancer risk management** *(cont.)*
>
> • To support this approach, an informed choice information initiative would be developed to assist men with understanding risk reduction for prostate cancer. This was subsequently launched in 2002 (NHS Cancer Screening Programmes, Prostate Cancer Risk Management 2006).

This compromise policy was necessary because of the widespread belief that a cancer test for men could not possibly fail to be beneficial. The principle of denying an intervention on the basis of evidence was not the problem, for the NHS has many examples of restrictions aimed at limiting ineffective and inefficient practices. The problem rested with the inability to accept the evidence as valid, because it ran so counter to belief. Our diagram now needs a fourth circle (Fig. 8.3).

The policy of allowing PSA testing for men who request it has been criticized because it ignores the evidence (Donovan *et al.* 2001; Law 2004), and subsequent research has added to concerns about the value of PSA screening (Stamey *et al.* 2004). The number of men in England receiving PSA tests and subsequent treatment grew sharply (Oliver *et al.* 2003), but is now showing signs of levelling off (Harling *et al.* 2005). Most of the men treated as a result of PSA screening are remaining free of cancer, which is no surprise given that most of them have been treated for a condition that would never have caused them a problem (see Fig. 7.1, p. 186). More than half of those treated suffer complications, most notably long-term incontinence or

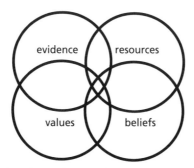

Fig. 8.3 Factors in policy making: evidence, resources, values and beliefs.

impotence (Potosky *et al.* 2000). In an attempt to try and reduce these ill effects, a range of alternatives to radical surgery or radiotherapy are being developed, involving laser, microwaves, extreme cold or implanted radioactive seeds. Whether any of the treatments are superior is unknown. One option for reducing treatment side effects is to opt for no intervention unless there is a significant rise in PSA levels; this is known as active monitoring. A major trial in the UK called the ProtecT study (University of Bristol ProtecT Study 2006) is comparing outcome in men with screen-detected cancer randomly allocated to either surgery, radiotherapy or active monitoring.

Many of the case studies in this book relate to cancer, which is no surprise given that many of the lessons learned in screening come from this field. It would, however, be a mistake to assume that other fields will be free of the uncertainties inherent in cancer screening. To emphasize this, it is worth looking at a case study from the field of genetics.

Case 8.7 Case study—genetic testing without consent and without benefit

In November 2000, the *British Medical Journal* published an article by Professor David Weatherall, founder of Oxford University's Institute of Molecular Medicine, based on a lecture given at the Millenium Festival of Medicine (Weatherall 2000).

The article describes, with great clarity, some of the many puzzles still to be unravelled in genetic medicine. Weatherall illustrates how, even for single gene disorders, the presence of a gene mutation does not automatically mean that the clinical disorder will be present.

For example:

- β-Thalassaemia is an inherited single gene disorder affecting haemoglobin synthesis. It leads to severe anaemia and other related effects.

- Amongst people who are homozygous for β-thalassaemia, some have very severe illness, some have only mild anaemia and some have no symptoms at all.

Case 8.7 Case study—genetic testing without consent and without benefit *(cont.)*

- Amongst people who are heterozygous for β-thalassaemia, some have no symptoms, yet others have severe illness comparable with that of homozygous cases.
- Sometimes siblings with identical inherited β-thalassaemia mutations have very different degrees of illness.

The implication of this is that other genes, and environmental factors, must play a part. It means that abnormal gene test results do not give certain information about the clinical condition even in single gene disorders, and that diagnosis and advice for affected families must be carried out by appropriately trained staff. If this is the case for single gene disorders, then the uncertainties are even greater for complex gene disorders (see Chapter 2, p. 52). For complex gene disorders, risk variants of genes are common in the population, and the implications of test results in any individual are completely unknown. Weatherall concludes that:

> ... the clinical application of new knowledge about the genome to common multigenic disorders may be slow. Relating genotype to phenotype is thus the challenge for genetic medicine over the next century (Weatherall 2000).

Advertising and sale of genetic tests for screening healthy people is available through the Internet, and there is considerable scope for testing that does no good and much harm. Given Weatherall's cautious words, you might think it reasonable only to test people with their informed consent, and where there is at least some possibility of benefit for the individual. This was not, however, the view taken by the prestigious scientific journal *Nature*, in an editorial published in 1995 (Anonymous 1995). The editorial asserted that it was wrong to insist on the patient's consent for predictive genetic testing, and argued that need for consent was:

> disputable in the now-novel circumstances; should a physician be hampered in providing the best care for a patient genetically susceptible to heart disease by the patient's wish not to know the genetic facts of his or her life? (Anonymous 1995).

The article went on to say that testing should be carried out irrespective of whether there was any therapeutic or prophylactic

> **Case 8.7 Case study—genetic testing without consent and without benefit** *(cont.)*
>
> remedy, or reproductive choice, arising from the results of testing. Testing should be done, so the anonymous writer argued, because:
>
> > wider genetic self-awareness will help bring about the more rational attitude towards the inevitability of death of which modern societies (and health-care systems) are in great need (Anonymous 1995).
>
> In other words, the author was saying that physicians should perform genetic tests on everyone no matter what resources this would need, irrespective of whether any benefit could ensue and without informed consent from the patient.

The editorial pre-dated Weatherall's talk by 5 years, and perhaps calmer voices are prevailing as time goes by. However, what the views in *Nature* illustrate is the strength of belief that clinical application of new technology and new tests must be a good thing, and must be used, just because they are there.

The importance of commercial interests

Companies with a market interest can get frustrated if screening is not adopted as quickly as they, and their shareholders, would like. They use all kinds of strategies to promote sales of medical products. These include funding of conferences and scientific meetings, provision of ghostwriters to get positive findings published quickly, suppression of publication of negative findings, direct lobbying of government, funding of patient pressure groups, assisting patient advocates with appeals against policy decisions and use of public relations firms to engineer a steady trickle of good news stories featuring individual cases claiming to have been helped by the technology. In the trade, the techniques that involve pressure groups and patient advocates are known as 'astroturfing' and 'guerilla marketing' because they successfully create the impression that the lobbying is coming purely from grassroots opinion and not from the industry. As the story below illustrates, it may be very difficult even for experienced medical editors to spot that the information they are being presented with is actually direct advertising.

Case 8.8 Case study—celebrity selling

In October 2001 a news item in the *British Medical Journal* (Watson 2001) featured a photograph of Jilly Cooper, Honor Blackman and Carol Smillie, all well-known celebrities in the UK. They were apparently actively campaigning on behalf of an organization known as European Women for HPV testing, with the aim of getting testing for human papilloma virus (HPV) adopted as the primary method of cervical screening within all 15 European Union states. The news article, entitled 'European women's group calls for human papillomavirus testing' included the following statements:

- A pan-European group of high profile women is pressing for introduction of routine testing for HPV in all 15 European Union states
- No European woman need die from cervical cancer
- The primary screening evidence (for HPV testing) is now overwhelming
- British members of the organization include authors, actresses, television personalities and politicians.

The then editor of the *BMJ*, Richard Smith, who usually took a robust approach to challenging manipulation by the pharmaceutical and equipment industry, made reference to the news item and to the promise of HPV testing in his 'Editor's Choice' column in the 6 October 2001 issue of the journal. In relation to conventional cytology, he noted that 'Perhaps the (cervical screening) test has been oversold. Doctors should spell out the difficulties of much of what they do ...', then went on to add '... it might be that testing for human papillomavirus infection would be much more effective—see the news item on page 772'. Smith presumably believed that this was a properly researched news story, rather than a carefully

Case 8.8 Case study—celebrity selling *(cont.)*

crafted advertisement produced on behalf of the test manufacturers. In fact the evidence at that time suggested that compared with the standards achieved by conventional cytology in the UK, HPV testing would make no measurable difference to deaths prevented and would increase the number of women harmed from overdetection (Woodman *et al.* 2001), it would worsen the harm from screening because of the stigmatization women feel when told they have a sexually transmitted virus for which there is no treatment (Maissi *et al.* 2004) and it would increase very substantially the costs of the programme (Raffle 1998) unless it fully replaced other screening methods.

In 2004 Anthony Barnett, an experienced journalist, was contacted by one of the celebrities who had been written to by European Women for HPV Testing. He did some proper investigative journalism (Barnett 2004) and discovered that:

♦ The European Womens' Group only existed as a PO Box address in Brussels, and staff at the post office would not disclose the PO Box owner.

♦ None of the celebrity backers that he contacted had heard of the group, despite being named on its website.

♦ By tracking down the signatory on a letter to one of the celebrities, he discovered that the campaign was run by Burson-Marsteller, one of the worlds largest public relations firms.

♦ Burson-Marsteller was working on behalf of Digene the manufacturers of the HPV test.

♦ Jeremy Galbraith, Chief Executive of Burson-Marsteller, said that the campaign was only about raising awareness of the links between HPV and cancer. This was despite the fact that the group was actively lobbying for the Hybrid Capture II test to be adopted for primary screening in all 15 European Union states.

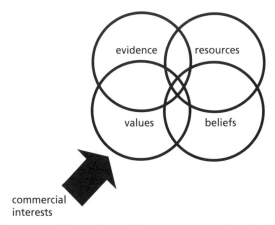

Fig. 8.4 Factors in policy making: evidence, resources, values, beliefs and commercial interests.

It is not unusual for governments to be influenced by this type of lobbying. They may be misled into thinking that pressure is genuinely coming from public opinion, or they may be well aware that the lobbyists are looking after the financial interests of the industry. The pharmaceutical and medical equipment industry can wield huge power by threatening to cut jobs in one country and relocate abroad. Politicians seldom take policy decisions solely on the basis of health. Employment and the economy are usually more important. So, our diagram now looks like Fig. 8.4.

What is a 'political' decision?

Maureen Roberts was the clinical director of the Edinburgh Breast Screening Project, one of four centres that pioneered breast screening in the UK. She was a lead researcher in the UK evaluation of breast screening. In June 1989 she died of breast cancer. In an article written shortly before her death, she reflected on the effects of screening, and on why the government was prepared to fund breast screening in preference to taking tobacco control seriously. Her article was published in the *British Medical Journal* in November 1989 and is well worth reading. Regarding the decision by the Forrest Committee, she says:

> It was clearly a matter of politics, a decision taken in an election year and now out of perspective.

She also describes, in a way that many of us involved in screening at that time will recognize as accurate, how the people delivering the service were reluctant to voice doubts:

> There is an air of evangelism, few people questioning what is actually being done. Are we brainwashing ourselves into thinking that we are making a dramatic impact on a serious disease before we brainwash the public? Many thousands of women will be invited for screening and those who attend are said to be 'compliant'. The compliance rate is not very high and I wonder what plans are being made to try and raise it. I hope very much that pressure is not put on women to attend. The decision must be theirs, and a truthful account of the facts must be made available to the public and the individual patient. It will not be what they want to hear (Roberts 1989).

Governments are elected to deliver what the people want. People believe that screening will harmlessly eliminate disease and pay for itself by reducing the need for treatment. The wise politician, who only thinks as far as surviving the next election (or even the next week in a ministerial post), inevitably makes decisions that match what the people believe in. Our challenge, and it is a considerable one, is to communicate and advocate public health evidence and values through the mass media (Chapman 2006) so that public opinions come closer to our evidence-based view of the world.

The ethics of policy making

Even with sound evidence of benefit and harm, and adequate information about resources, the policy maker's task still involves difficult judgements. We have already looked at how people's beliefs about screening (see p. 235) and strongly held values within society (see p. 231) can challenge the policy maker's rational approach to decision taking. However, there are even more reasons for difficulty. This is because when you are weighing up conflicting needs and aims, there is no single 'right' policy. Ethical theory can help to clarify the principles on which decisions may be based, and the proper processes that should be followed, but this still does not make the decisions simple.

Dilemmas can be faced within each type of policy decision (we listed the types of decision on p. 217). To illustrate this, we can look at the implications of some of the main ethical frameworks and principles used to help with health policy decisions, namely:

+ Utilitarianism
+ Quality adjusted life years
+ Autonomy
+ Justice
+ Human rights
+ Accountability and right of appeal

Utilitarianism

One way of looking at health policy decisions is to ask which course of action will produce maximum welfare or benefit. This approach is known as 'consequential' because it judges the merit of a course of action not by examining the action itself, but by examining its consequences. A utilitarian approach means using society's resources as efficiently as possible to increase 'good' for humankind. Immediately one can see that there are problems:

+ There are all kinds of measures that could be chosen for weighing up welfare or benefit—you might be interested in well-being, happiness and social 'good'. How do you tell how well you are doing? Inevitably length of life is the easiest to measure.

+ Provided that there is a net benefit overall, the efficiency equation tends to disregard the harm, even death, suffered by some.

+ The most efficient course of action may deny any help to certain categories of people, and this conflicts directly with principles of social justice.

Box 8.2 Utilitarianism

Jeremy Bentham lived from 1748 to 1832. He and his followers, the Benthamites, launched the idea of utilitarianism. The most enduring description of its principles is probably John Stuart Mill's 1861 publication of the same name, which contains the now famous phrase 'the greatest good for the greatest number'. The utilitarians held that actions should be judged by their consequences for

Box 8.2 Utilitarianism *(cont.)*

human benefit, measured in terms of human happiness. They advocated the welfare of the many, in reaction to the often oppressive social control exerted by the Church, either directly or through the State, and the harmful consequences this could have for ordinary citizens. The utilitarian philosophy did not advocate imposition of actions just because they could bring good, it was more that they emphasized outcome as a means of judging whether something was right. In John Stuart Mill's famous 1859 publication *On liberty*, he argues the principle, highly relevant to public health policy, that the state has no right to impose interventions on the individual even if this is ostensibly for their own good.

The struggle actually to measure beneficial consequences dates back to at least 1799 when the economist Sir John Sinclair called for a means to measure 'a quantum of human happiness'.

One result of a utilitarian approach to screening has been a tendency to weigh up the benefit and harm as a simple equation:

(deaths prevented) – (deaths caused from complications) = net deaths prevented

This leads to the setting of targets for high uptake on the grounds that this will bring the greatest benefit to public health. Individual family doctors, programme leads and screening managers are then rewarded or penalized according to whether uptake targets are met. The best way of achieving high uptake is to give unbalanced information, stressing the benefit and glossing over the harm. So the simple arithmetic that tells you screening can be unhesitatingly recommended because of the net benefit, is hiding an important moral dilemma, memorably illustrated in Dostoyevsky's *The brothers Karamazov*. In the novel, one of the brothers, Ivan Karamazov, aggressively challenges his more pious brother Aloysha on his desire to improve the lot of mankind, by asking him to say whether he would sanction the mistreatment of one innocent child if, by so doing, a greater number were saved. If Ivan Karamazov were attending the National Screening

Committee, he might ask if the committee members would be willing to shoot one person for the benefit of others. It is hard to counter the argument that there is no ethical difference between using a gun to kill someone you can see, and accepting that someone you cannot see will be killed as a result of your policy.

Coercion to achieve high uptake falls into the very trap that John Stuart Mill warned of in *On liberty*, and it rewards staff for imposing potentially harmful interventions, albeit for the best of reasons. The population is being treated as though it were a single patient, and the screening programme is being administered universally because it is in 'the patient's' interest. This ignores the fact that the patient in this case is made up of numerous individuals, each of whom has a right to autonomy (see below). Public health advocates need to be mindful of this, and the criticisms contained in books such as Skrabanek's *The death of humane medicine* should be compulsory reading for public health practitioners (Skrabanek 1994), however uncomfortable we may find this.

It may be that the tendency to adopt a coercive approach in screening stems from its close association, administratively and conceptually, with public health programmes for communicable disease control. Communicable disease control can involve immunization, mass screening, contact screening, isolation and quarantine. However, there are crucial differences between programmes aimed at preventing epidemics and programmes aimed at reducing risk for individuals:

- With immunization, everyone potentially gains because all could contract the infection if there were no immunization programme. With screening, most people do not benefit as most people would not get the disease. The 'protective effect of a negative test' sometimes quoted by statisticians is, as Knox pointed out, a flawed concept (Knox 1991). Negative tests are predictive, like an engineer's survey saying your house is sound, but they do not protect.

- With immunization, high uptake is essential to achieve herd immunity, and all are at greater risk if uptake is low. With screening, high uptake may be more economically efficient if it gets the best return from fixed resources, but the benefit is in direct proportion to the uptake, and the benefit to the individual is determined by his or her individual choice about participation.

- With infectious disease control, the individual has a duty not to endanger other members of the public, and public health legislation confers powers on the state for enforcing this duty. With screening, the individual is free to make their own choice and has no duty to comply.

The other comparison with immunization is strangely paradoxical:

- Successful immunization makes infections rare, and once they are beyond living memory the public are more aware of harm—often imagined harm—from immunization, than they are of the benefit. Maintenance of high immunization rates may therefore need publicity about the continued threat of infectious epidemics. In contrast, successful screening reduces serious disease only marginally and often increases the number of apparent cases because of overdiagnosis, so public perception of the threat of disease stays high. The harm is unrecognized because of the popularity paradox (see p. 68).

Quality-adjusted life years

The health economist Alan Williams, and his colleagues at York University, promoted the concept of the 'quality-adjusted life year (QALY)' in UK circles (Williams 1985), although it was first developed in the USA. It provides a method of comparing value for money of different interventions by computing the benefit in terms of years of life, adjusted according to the quality of life achieved. It is a valuable concept, but there are dangers in viewing it as the total answer to resource allocation problems:

- It is extremely difficult to define valid weightings for quality of life that would be generally agreed upon by all potential recipients of treatment. Would we choose 1 year of life without pain, in preference to 2 years of life with pain, or with anxiety or with disability?

- Moral questions about how society should allocate resources become concealed within an apparently scientific equation, underpinned by a solely utilitarian approach irrespective of need or level of existing suffering.

- The end results of the health economic calculations are usually expressed as a single £ per QALY value, implying an accuracy that is an illusion. For example, a standard textbook contains the much quoted estimate that cervical screening costs £200 per quality-adjusted life year (Savulescu *et al.* 2003). Yet it requires 1000 women to be screened for 35 years to prevent one death from cervical cancer (Raffle *et al.* 2003). This QALY estimate is clearly wrong. If each woman has around seven tests during the 35 years, and even if the cost per test together with all the associated programme of activities that goes with testing is only £40, then the woman who has her life prolonged would need to avoid 1400 years of lost life to arrive at an estimate of £200.

Autonomy

In June 2000 the National Screening Committee for the UK retreated to Windsor Great Park for 2 days of seminars and discussions. This retreat was prompted by recognition that arguments about the content of information leaflets on screening could never be resolved until the matter of their purpose was clarified. The papers presented to the Committee were published in a special issue of the journal *Health Expectations* (Coulter 2001). The outcome of the Committee's deliberations was agreement that:

> the purpose of information about screening is to allow individuals to make an informed choice about whether to participate (National Screening Committee 2000).

Before June 2000 the implicit policy had been that the purpose of information about screening was to encourage attendance.

The arguments about the contents of the leaflets were prompted by continued questioning, predominantly from staff within the screening programmes, of the traditional approach to information giving. The traditional approach was to give very simple and persuasive messages about screening, implying that screening gave certain protection and had no adverse consequences. The basis for this questioning of current practice related to the following factors:

- By encouraging people to accept screening either by appealing to their sense of duty, or by giving them overoptimistic expectations of the benefit and safety of screening, we were ignoring an important ethical principle, that of individual autonomy.

- The absence of any information about harms and limitations of screening meant that when people were let down by screening, they felt angry, sometimes to an extreme degree. This anger and disillusionment is in itself a harm, and some people would remain embittered long after the material health effects of the screening-related harm had ceased.

- By implying that screening was highly effective and capable of totally preventing a condition, we were causing patients, and the health service staff caring for them, to overlook signs and symptoms in the mistaken belief that a recent negative screening result ruled the condition out. This led to delayed diagnosis and to subsequent anger and bitterness.

- By overstating the effectiveness and simplicity of screening, we were creating an impossible working environment for screening staff, who would come under attack, often with high profile press coverage, for 'blunders' and 'failure' even where screening had been conducted to high standards.

- By overstating and oversimplifying the benefits of screening and failing to explain harms and limitations, we were creating a mythology around screening that made it difficult to achieve rational policy making and reasonable legal judgements.

So the case for giving balanced information was practical as well as ethical, but the autonomy argument is important in its own right. If we ignore autonomy, we are imposing harm on uninformed participants.

Autonomy applies to adults but not children. The principle of autonomy does not mean that all actions by an individual must be free from constraint. Autonomous individuals are constrained, for example, by laws prohibiting driving on the wrong side of the road, by duties to their employer saying they will turn up to work and by the limits of their own resources. Autonomy means that it is up to an

Box 8.3 Definition of autonomy

The ethical principle that independent actions and choices of an individual should not be constrained by others.

individual whether, for example, they smoke (provided they do not expose others to second-hand smoke), whether they take recommended medication and whether they undergo screening.

The General Medical Council for the UK gives guidance to doctors clearly stating that autonomy must be respected.

The practical and ethical reasons for giving full information, as opposed to information designed solely to encourage attendance, are powerful, but there are also strong arguments that weigh in the other direction, and until 2000 these were the arguments that determined the national approach. These arguments against giving balanced information are:

♦ There is a risk that uptake will decrease and therefore overall benefit will fall. There is a danger that it could be that those at highest risk with most to gain from screening will be the ones to stay away. There is, however, no evidence that information is more important than accessibility in ensuring equity of uptake across risk groups.

♦ More staff time is needed in order to ensure that participants understand what the programme is for and what the benefits and limitations are.

Box 8.4 General Medical Council Guidance (General Medical Council 1998)

You must respect patients' autonomy … their right to decide whether or not to undergo any medical intervention, even where a refusal may result in harm to themselves.

The guidance warns against assuming that apparent compliance constitutes informed consent.

Specifically relating to screening the advice states:

you must ensure that anyone considering whether to consent to screening can make a proper informed decision …. You should be careful to explain clearly the purpose of screening; the likelihood of positive/negative findings and possibility of false-positive/false-negative results; the uncertainties and risks attached to the screening process and any significant medical, social or financial implications.

- If full information led to very low uptake such that a service is barely viable, then cost-effectiveness would be diminished.

The policy decision taken by the UK National Screening Committee was that the purpose of information about screening is to ensure informed choice. This means that the practical challenges of training staff to help people make an informed choice, and of developing easy to understand, balanced information and making it widely available, are now beginning to be tackled.

Justice

In the section about utilitarianism (see p. 245) we mentioned that choosing policy based only on efficiency may run counter to principles of justice, if for example some groups get no chance of benefit.
Justice is about what is right, morally good and fair.

- Criminal justice is concerned with redress and punishment when one citizen wrongs another.

- Social justice is about the freedoms of each individual in society – to be represented in government, to think, say and meet with others as they choose, and so on.

- Distributive justice is about allocation of goods or utilities within a society. Two main approaches are either to distribute according to capacity to benefit, this is termed 'end-state theory', or to distribute according to entitlement, this is termed 'entitlement theory'. End-state theory will judge the needy as most deserving of resources. Entitlement theory looks at the transactions that have led to the current distribution and judges anyone who has behaved lawfully and reasonably as entitled to equivalent resource.

Distributive justice is relevant to screening policy when decisions are being made about:

- Whether to invest resources in screening or into other interventions instead

- Who should be eligible and who should be invited for any given programme

- How much extra resources should be invested to reach hard to reach groups, such as different cultural and ethnic groups, those with visual impairment, learning difficulty or physical disability.

There is no certain way of deciding what is fair. John Rawls, who lived from 1921 to 2002, wrote extensively about social justice, and his proposals have been highly influential in recent times (Rawls 1971). One of the concepts that Rawls put forward was that we should choose rules to create a society we would be comfortable with whatever our place in it. He called this the 'veil of ignorance'. It requires us to imagine that we are going to have to live in a society, but we do not know whether we will be born into it male or female, rich or poor, healthy or ill. Rawls argues that we should choose rules that would make us equally comfortable to live in that society whether we were ill and disadvantaged, or whether we were healthy and affluent.

Our experience with consulting members of the public about screening, though we have no data to back this up, suggests that many people place a value on ensuring wide access to the possibility of benefit, even if that means diluting the actual magnitude of benefit. It emphasizes the importance of 'the greatest number' element of the utilitarian principle (see p. 245) and means that a simple algebraic approach is misleading. An extra 1 year of life for 20 people is likely to be judged preferable to 25 years of extra life for one person. This is consistent with the actual experiences of countries that have attempted to make cervical screening more cost-effective by targeting it to those most at risk (Wilkinson *et al.* 1992). The targeting tends to be viewed by the public as illogical and discriminatory.

So, if there are sound reasons for choosing age restrictions, as for example with breast screening under 50 where this does more harm than good (see p. 232), then time and effort are needed for communicating these reasons to the public, and for continuing to communicate them over time. If we do not, then the obvious message to the ordinary man or woman in the street is that the policy is unfair.

Deciding entitlement to services purely on the grounds of age, gender, race, ethnicity, religion, sexual orientation, class, education, economic status, disability or health is seen as contrary to the principles of social justice. This does not mean that age cut-offs, or screening offered selectively to certain ethnic groups, cannot ever be justified. Certain age groups may be at very low risk so harm will outweigh benefit; certain ethnic groups may be at high risk so are the only group where screening is beneficial. It simply means that the eligibility criteria must be demonstrably derived from evidence about risk and capacity to benefit.

There have been cases where the UK courts have adjudicated on matters relating to funding decisions in healthcare, although no cases to date have related to decisions about screening policy. The courts have acknowledged that painful decisions about resource allocation are necessary, and that it is the duty of health service staff, and not of the courts, to take these decisions (UK Clinical Ethics Network 2004). The legal scrutiny focuses on whether the decisions had been taken lawfully, for example did the decision taker have the power to take the decision, were correct procedures followed, were relevant considerations taken into account and was the decision reasonable and proportionate.

Human rights

In 1998 the European Convention on Human Rights was incorporated into UK Law by the passing of the Human Rights Act. The European Convention was drawn up after the Second World War, to guard against the human rights violations enacted by the Nazis. The Convention contains several articles that have implications for healthcare policy.

+ Article two states there is a 'right to life'.
+ Article eight provides a right to respect for private and family life.
+ Article fourteen prohibits discrimination.

Since 1998 many have wondered if the 'right to life' will be interpreted by courts of law as meaning that all interventions in healthcare must be provided. It seems more likely, however, that UK and European courts will steer clear of judging Article two in terms of a right to interventions that lengthen life, as opposed to freedom from interventions that actively threaten life. There is a distinction between basic human rights (such as freedom of speech, freedom of movement, freedom from persecution) and tax-funded services (such as liver transplants, cancer drugs or screening programmes). The courts will no doubt be acutely aware that if they uphold the rights of individual

A to have an expensive treatment, then they can be challenged by individual B who claims that their right to life is infringed because resources have all been used up on individual A.

Accountability and right of appeal

All countries struggle with setting fair policy in a world where no budget could possibly fund everything that medicine is capable of. In every nation, governments and commercial sector organizations design mechanisms that ration resources in ways that seem compatible with the values of a particular society. Norman Daniels, Professor of Philosophy from Tufts University, and James Sabin, Professor of Psychiatry at Harvard, describe some principles for assuring accountability in a democratic society, through the use of processes that accentuate fairness and openness (Daniels and Sabin 1997, 1998). Part of their thesis stems from the fact that in the USA much of the decision taking by commercial 'health plan' providers is governed by 'market accountability', and this accountability leaves many consumers objecting to the restrictions on care and questioning their reasonableness. Daniels and Sabin argue that a different kind of accountability is needed, and they call this 'accountability for reasonableness'. They highlight four key conditions for ethical decision taking:

- ◆ Publicity condition. Decisions and their rationale must be publicly accessible.

- ◆ Relevance condition. The rationale for decisions must rest on evidence, reasons and principles that all 'fair-minded' parties (managers, clinicians, patients and consumers in general) can agree are relevant to deciding appropriate patient care under necessary resource constraints. 'Fair-minded' is taken to mean people who seek to co-operate with others on terms that are mutually justifiable.

- ◆ Appeals condition. There is a mechanism for challenge and dispute resolution.

- ◆ Enforcement condition. There is either voluntary or public regulation of the process to ensure that the first three conditions are met.

This gives a useful guide for policy makers. It means that decisions must be taken openly, reasonably and lawfully, processes must be properly documented and there must be a mechanism for appeals to be heard. Within the NHS at the moment, accountability for most resource allocation decisions rests locally with the Primary Care Trusts. For others it rests centrally with the National Institute for Health and Clinical Excellence, and there is a muddle of contradictory advice and directives, and appeal mechanisms, overlaying the whole picture (Raffle 2006). The accountability for decision taking on screening policy is clear, and rests with the National Screening Programmes. Policy will never be simple or right, and it will always need to evolve as new evidence emerges and as society changes. Clear central accountability provides a foundation on which to build quality and reasonableness.

To conclude

So here we are at the end of the book, and nearly 150 years since Horace Dobell wrote of his ambition to empty the hospital waiting rooms and cut the enormous expenditure on drugs. The ambition remains. Our knowledge of the difficulties associated with Dobell's proposed solution has grown substantially. Key achievements are:

◆ Fifty years ago the idea of conducting a randomized controlled trial to measure the impact of early detection in healthy people was regarded by most people as unethical—how could you randomize people to receive only usual care? Now it is widely recognized that without carefully conducted controlled trials we risk imposing harm for no benefit, as happened with infant screening for neuroblastoma.

◆ Thirty years ago the idea of acknowledging harm or limitations, or of explaining these to potential participants, was regarded as highly unacceptable. This could not happen, it was argued, because it risked 'undermining the programme'. Uptake was the sole performance measure. Now the giving of balanced information is an essential component of offering good quality risk reduction to the public.

◆ Forty years ago the idea of taking 5 or 10 years to plan and implement a national programme would have been regarded as unjustified bureaucratic delay. Now it is recognized that if a programme is worthwhile, then it has to be delivered to a high quality if it is to achieve its potential benefit. This takes time and resources for training and implementation.

◆ Twenty years ago the suggestion that pathology found in symptomless people might be inconsequential was greeted with derision. Now there are books published for the general public explaining the overdiagnosis problem.

We are already noticing a difference in the understanding of these concepts amongst people under 25, who have grown up in a world where debate about harm and benefit has been the norm. Our teaching sessions with medical students now are a very different experience from 10 and 20 years ago.

The challenge is to develop ways of researching, and offering high quality and affordable risk reduction for the twenty-first century society. As with so many things, the more we learn about health and illness, the more we find what we do not know. One of the biggest threats is the commercial incentive to offer tests and remedies to the worried well, whether this will be beneficial or not. Another is the tendency to assume that intervention in healthy people must always be better than leaving things alone.

Summary points

The way that screening policy is made and enacted varies widely from country to country. It ranges from central policy making and national provision, through to national recommendations, with the onus on individuals to procure screening from independent providers.

Policy decisions are concerned with whether and how to start a programme, whether actively to stop a screening activity from starting, whether to change tests, frequency, eligible groups, etc. within an existing programme, how much central control to exert over quality assurance and what information to make available to participants.

Four main factors that influence screening policy are evidence, resources, values and beliefs. Commercial factors also play a part.

The UK National Screening Committee Criteria provide a logical framework for approaching policy decisions, but very few screening programmes actually meet all the criteria and it is seldom possible to follow an entirely logical approach.

Summary points *(cont.)*

Evidence for policy making must be valid and presented in a way that makes it as easy as possible to understand. It must be appropriately framed and balanced. The right questions must be asked about costs, and these must be set in the context of the whole programme of healthcare.

When evidence points to a policy that conflicts with the values or beliefs of the society, the likelihood is that the values and beliefs will have the strongest influence.

Commercial companies use a wide range of methods, including 'third party techniques' and 'celebrity selling' to influence policy makers and the general public in favour of screening.

Politicians inevitably make decisions that reflect what the public believe in and want. The challenge for public health is to use mass communication and advocacy so that public opinions come closer to our evidence-based view of the world.

Decisions about screening policy bring ethical dilemmas. Utilitarian principles might suggest that harm, even death, for some individuals can be overlooked if a greater number benefit. The principle of autonomy requires that information about harm be made available even if this discourages people from attending. Justice requires that no one is discriminated against, and that the needy receive a service. Human rights and legal requirements demand that decisions are made lawfully, accountably, reasonably and with right of appeal.

National, rather than local, policy making has the best chance of fulfilling the requirements for valid scrutiny of evidence and resources, due process, transparency, fairness, accountability and right of appeal.

Test yourself

Question one

For each of the following terms, write down an explanation and illustrate with an example:

(a) Natural frequencies

(b) Framing

(c) Balance.

Question two

Imagine you have been brought in to assist a national group that is preparing information to assist policy makers in formulating recommendations about routine testing for rare genetic conditions in all newborn babies.

♦ Technology is available (tandem mass spectrometry) that means many tests could be added routinely to the existing newborn bloodspot examination. Currently only phenylketonuria and congenital hypothyroidism are tested for.

♦ The group has received information from the equipment manufacturers saying that 87 conditions can accurately be detected.

♦ The group has received information from advocacy groups supporting the introduction of screening.

♦ The group believes there will be minimal costs associated with introducing screening for the new conditions because the bloodspot tests are already being taken, and the laboratories already have the necessary technology to do these extra tests.

♦ Several authoritative articles have stated the opinion that screening will be beneficial.

On the basis of this information, the group is already writing its report for the policy makers. They are recommending that testing be introduced routinely for some 30–50 conditions.

The following statements relate to the interpretation of the above information. Which do you agree with?

(a) There can be no harm in recommending all the screening tests.

(b) The new tests must be beneficial because the test accuracy data look impressive.

(c) The conclusion that costs will be minimal is wrong.

(d) It is safe to assume that positive cases will benefit from early detection.

(e) Because some laboratories are doing the tests already, there is no alternative to adding all the screening, as the present situation is inequitable.

(f) The policy making process is reasonable because it has included input from advocacy groups.

(g) An independently conducted systematic review of all the available evidence on benefit and harm from routine testing for the 87 rare conditions should be commissioned.

(h) The information prepared so far by the group is sufficient for the policy decision because the group has kept good records of its meetings and discussions.

(i) There is no point challenging the adequacy of the report prepared by the group because newspaper articles are already arguing that the testing must be introduced, and several politicians are backing the introduction of the new tests.

(j) There will be harm from screening when treatment is given to babies positive on testing but who would have remained healthy.

(k) Uncertain results, and cases undetected by the screening, will not be a problem.

Question three

Which of the following statements are true:

(a) John Stuart Mill argued that it was acceptable to impose things on people for their own good, whether they liked it or not.

(b) Utilitarianism is about improving the welfare of the community.

(c) There is an ethical difference between the act of causing direct harm to an individual, versus enacting a policy that will lead to harm.

(d) The ethical principle that says an individual's actions and choices should not be constrained by others is known as 'individualism'.

(e) In the UK, national policy states that the information about screening should be designed for encouraging high uptake.

(f) It is against the law to have age restrictions on access to screening.

(g) End-state theories of distributive justice argue that those most needy should get more resource devoted to them than those without the same level of need.

(h) Rawl's 'veil of ignorance' theory says that the fairest way of distributing resources is to make decisions in secret.

(i) When health policy decisions have been challenged in the courts, the judgements made have related more to whether decisions were made lawfully and without discrimination, rather than the actual decision.

Answers

Chapter 1

Question one

Statements a, c, f, and g were not amongst the concerns raised by the rationalists in the 1960s. All the rest were.

Question two

Features in the early days of cervical screening in the UK:

No consistent policy about who should be screened or how often.

No system for inviting all eligible people at regular intervals.

No training or quality assurance for sample takers or sample readers.

No consistent classification system for abnormalities on cytology.

Mainly the low risk women attended, as they were more likely to know about the service and use it.

Treatment of screen-detected abnormality was not regarded as anything to do with the screening service.

Treatments (if they happened) were very invasive with side effects.

Very simplistic information was given to participants, resulting in anger and disillusionment for women who felt let down by screening.

There was a lack of definitive evidence that screening caused more good than harm.

No national co-ordination.

No planned approach to research and development relating to potential advances in screening.

Features of the UK cervical screening programme in the late 1990s:

Strong national co-ordination team drawing on expertise from throughout the programme.

Nationally directed research and development for potential advances in screening.

National policy uniformly applied.

Reliable call and recall system based on population registers and using national software.

Uniform mandatory training and proficiency testing for sample takers and sample readers.

Uniform classification system and routine scrutiny of performance statistics for individuals and laboratories.

Service accessible and publicized to all.

Treatment services included in the quality assurance systems, with failsafe arrangements to ensure that treatment happens when needed.

Less invasive treatments with fewer side effects.

Balanced information explaining the limitations as well as the benefits, and offering informed choice.

Evidence from UK cervical cancer death rates shows a definite change in the age-specific pattern in cohorts born since the 1930s, and the key outcomes good and bad have been acknowledged, and quantified.

Chapter 2

Question one

(a) This is screening. The woman has no symptoms and the implied promise is reduced risk of heart disease by finding things early. It is not being delivered as a programme—if she does have a positive result it will be up to her to arrange further investigations. Also, it is not based on sound evidence and it is definitely not recommended as a useful screening test (Gibbons *et al.* 2002). Question four at the end of Chapter 4 illustrates why.

(b) This is a safety check. Although this man has no symptoms of heart disease, he is having the test to help ensure a safe anaesthetic the next day, rather than to reduce his risk of heart disease.

(c) This is a test for infection control. The man has no symptoms of TB but is a contact of a known case. The reason for testing him is partly to help him with prompt treatment if he is infected, and partly to control the spread of the communicable disease. Contact tracing tests do have some similarities to the types of screening that we are focusing on in this book, but there are also important differences.

(d) This is a diagnostic test.

(e) This is screening. The man has no symptoms, and he hopes the test will reduce his risk of dying of prostate cancer. It is not being delivered as part of a quality-assured programme. Also, it is not based on sound evidence that benefit outweighs harm.

(f) This is screening. The woman has no symptoms, and the aim of testing is to reduce her risk of dying of breast cancer. It is being delivered as a quality-assured programme. In most breast screening programmes there is no upper age limit for the eligible group, although routine invitations are not usually issued beyond 70 because it is more practical to allow healthy older women to opt in.

(g) This is a safety check. The man has no symptoms of liver disease, but the test gives a baseline from which to check if any liver damage is occurring, and ensures that the drug is not given if he already has compromised liver function.

(h) This is for the protection of others.

(i) This is testing for an associated condition. Use of a screening test would be inadequate, he needs a diagnostic test.

Question two

The answer depends on what programmes you chose, but here are some examples. Please note that the eligible groups, and the tests used, will vary from place to place. This is because many decisions about precisely how to deliver screening are based on judgements about relative cost and effectiveness. The main purpose of this question is to get you thinking about what precisely is involved in any screening programme. All too often one hears or reads discussion about screening with little clarity over the steps involved.

Aortic aneurysm screening

(a) men at age 65

(b) abdominal ultrasound

(c) possibly CT scan, or possibly no further investigation

(d) elective surgical repair of abdominal aortic aneurysm

(e) reduced risk of death from ruptured aortic aneurysm.

Congenital hypothyroidism

(a) all newborn babies

(b) heelprick bloodspot test on newborn baby to test for thyroid stimulating hormone

(c) further blood tests to measure thyroxine levels (T_4) and possibly a thyroid scan in some cases

(d) oral administration of thyroid hormone

(e) reduced risk of mental impairment.

Sight-threatening diabetic retinopathy

(a) all insulin-dependent diabetics

(b) visual inspection of digital photograph of retina

(c) more detailed visual inspection of retina, with magnification, performed by an experienced opthalmologist

(d) laser treatment of new vessel formation

(e) reduced risk of sight impairment.

Cervical screening

(a) women aged 25–64 with a cervix

(b) visual microscopic inspection of cells from cervix (cytology)

(c) visual inspection of cervix with magnification (colposcopy) and visual microscopic inspection of tissue sample (histology)

(d) destruction or excision of abnormal tissue

(e) reduced risk of death from cancer of the cervix.

Chapter 3

Question one

A positive screening test result is finding an aneurysm that is at suffi-cient risk of rupture to warrant offer of elective surgery. This is usually defined as an aneurysm of at least 50 or 55 mm diameter.

A negative screening test result is no aneurysm. An aneurysm is defined as a widening of the aorta to at least one and a half times its usual width, so a negative result is an aortic diameter less than one and a half times the usual.

The uncertain test result is where someone has an aorta bigger than one and a half times the usual diameter, but smaller that 50 or 55 mm. In this group, the risk of surgery could outweigh the risk of rupture, but the aorta is not normal and the aneurysm might or might not expand. This group is advised to have repeat ultrasound examinations to see if there is any increase in size, usually annually for aneurysms less than 35 mm, six monthly for aneurysms 35–49 mm.

The intervention is elective surgery, i.e. planned as opposed to emergency, to repair the aneurysm.

The four subdivisions in the intervention group:

♦ Would have died of ruptured aneurysm without screening, and thanks to the elective surgery they either live longer and die of something else, or live longer but still die from rupturing their aneurysm.

♦ Would have ruptured their aneurysm without screening, but the leak would have been slow enough to allow for successful emergency surgery. With screening they have the surgery sooner, but the outcome is no different.

♦ Would have died of ruptured aneurysm without screening, still die of ruptured aneurysm despite elective repair, and with no lengthening of life.

♦ Would never have known that their aneurysm existed if they had not had screening. So screening has led to surgery that they did not need.

The complications and side effects for the intervention group include a risk of death from the anaesthetic and the surgery, and risk of surgical complications such as infection of the artificial artery, breakdown of the repair, deep vein thrombosis, pulmonary embolism, etc.

People who develop disease after negative results are the people who die of ruptured aneurysm after being given a negative screening result or an uncertain screening result not leading to intervention.

People who develop disease outside the eligible group are younger men, older men or women who die of ruptured aneurysm but were not in the eligible group for screening.

Question two

There is no right answer to this as it is about how you might feel. Research tells us that different individuals react very differently, and that often people feel a wide range of emotional reactions simultaneously. Common responses to a screen-detected diagnosis include anxiety about the implications (ranging from mild to extreme), relief that the condition has been found, and anger if there is little in the way of information and support. The information at the time a test is offered may not have prepared participants for any negative consequences. Focus groups drawn from the general population are sometimes consulted in drawing up information for participants. They tend to say that information about interventions, risks or uncertain categories of disease is off-putting and too detailed, and should not be included. People who do suffer ill effects give different views. They feel that information should mention all consequences, and that a passing mention of 'a small risk' is inadequate. A risk may be low, but it is hard to describe death as a 'small' risk.

Question three

(a) A

(b) B

(c) A

(d) A

(e) B

(f) B

(g) A

(h) B

(i) A

(j) B

Question four

For a programme with a minimum of undetected cases:

Advantages:

The programme will achieve maximum potential for avoiding deaths from ruptured aortic aneurysm.

Disadvantages:

There will be many people damaged by being told they need monitoring, and who may worry about their aneurysm and when it is going to rupture.

By operating on many aneurysms, the programme will cause complications and side effects in a significant number, and some fatalities.

There could be adverse publicity about surgical deaths in people whose aneurysms were relatively low risk

The programme will be relatively expensive, diverting resources from more beneficial activities

For a programme with minimum overdiagnosis and overtreatment:

Advantages:

There will be less damage to the healthy population as more people are correctly told they are negative.

Surgery will be performed in those most likely to benefit from it so the complications and side effects will be less compared with the benefit.

The programme will be relatively inexpensive.

Disadvantages:

Some people could feel they are being denied a service.

Some people may feel that more follow-up is needed in order to be 'safe'.

There could be adverse publicity about deaths in people who were screen negative.

Chapter 4

Question one

The control group and the intervention group have not been handled in exactly the same way in relation to inclusions, exclusions, and assignment of cause of death.

Inclusions. The intervention group includes only people registered with a family doctor, whereas the control group includes all residents in a defined geographical area. This introduces a potential bias as the control group includes homeless people, and other non-registered groups whereas the intervention group does not.

Exclusions. In the intervention group, all people who responded to the researchers' letter and who had existing lung cancer were excluded from the study. No such exclusion was applied in the control group, as there was no process of writing to the subjects and then assessing them. This introduces a bias, by excluding some of the lung cancer cases from the analysis.

Assignment of cause of death. In the intervention group, the case notes are scrutinized for each subject who dies, but case notes for deaths in the control group are not examined. Those scrutinizing the case notes will know that the person is in the offered screening group unless they are entirely ignorant of the study design. Both these factors add to the unreliability of the assignment of outcome. It is well known that case note scrutiny can lead to revision of the cause of death as assigned on the death certificate. For example, it may reveal that the primary site of the cancer is not the lung, or that co-existing illness such as heart disease was the actual cause of the death. Allowing the potential to revise the cause of death but only in the intervention group introduces bias.

A competent peer reviewer would point out these flaws to the editors and would advise that the findings of the study are biased and are likely to be unreliable.

Question two

(a) If prevalence is 5 per cent, then in 10 000 symptomless people there will be 500 (5/100 × 10 000) who have undiagnosed coronary heart disease.

(b) The first numbers you can fill in are the 10 000 total in the bottom right hand corner, the 500 total with coronary heart disease at the bottom of the left hand column, and the remainder which is 9500 without coronary heart disease in the bottom of the next column. Then you work out the true positives, which are 50 per cent of all the 500 with coronary heart disease, and the true negatives, which are 90 per cent of the 9500 without coronary heart disease. All the other boxes can be worked out by addition and subtraction. When you have finished, the numbers in your two by two table (using A B C D as in Table 4.1) are A 250, B 950, C 250, D 8 550. Column totals are 500 and 9500. Row totals are 1200 and 8800.

(c) A total of 950 have a positive result but no coronary heart disease.

(d) A total of 250 have a negative result but do have coronary heart disease.

(e) The positive predictive value is 250 out of 1200, which as a proportion is 0.2 and as a percentage is 20.8 per cent.

(f) Exercise ECG is not recommended for screening symptomless people because you subject a substantial number of people with no coronary heart disease (950 out of 10 000 screened) to invasive and potentially dangerous investigations (angiography) as a consequence of positive screening test results. It is uncertain whether you help any of those who you identify as having symptomless coronary heart disease. You falsely reassure half of the people who have symptomless coronary heart disease and this could lead to a greater likelihood of them subsequently ignoring symptoms or of ignoring advice about risky behaviour (smoking, inactivity, poor diet).

Question three

(a) This time the numbers in your two by two table are A 50, B 990, C 50, D 8 910. Column totals are 100 and 9900. Row totals are 1040 and 8960.

(b) Positive predictive value is 50/1 040 = 0.048, or expressing it as a percentage 4.8 per cent of those with positive results will actually have the condition

(c) When the prevalence was five per cent, the PPV was 250/1200 = 0.208, or expressing it as a percentage 20.8 per cent of those with positive results actually have the condition

(d) The same test has worse positive predictive value when it is used in a group with lower prevalence.

Question four

(a) The survival rate at 1 year is 20 per cent (20 alive out of 100) and the mortality is 80 per cent (80 dead out of 100).

(b) The survival rate at 1 year is 46.6 per cent (70 alive out of 150) and the mortality is 53.3 per cent (80 dead out of 150).

(c) The number dying from lung cancer each year has stayed the same at 80.

(d) The stage and grade at diagnosis will look substantially better when expressed as a percentage of all diagnosed lung cancers, because the screen-detected cancers will contain a high proportion of localized and slow growing cancers, some of which would never have become symptomatic and clinically important during the persons lifetime.

(e) This example is in essence the same as the neuroblastoma case study (p. 89). The appropriate conclusion from the data is that deaths have not changed, overdiagnosis and overtreatment are happening, and the apparent improvement in survival is the result of length time bias and overdiagnosis bias. Screening should not be recommended, and randomized controlled trials are needed if questions about benefit and harm are to be answered. Establishing rapport with the pressure group, and sensitively and diplomatically explaining your reservations without belittling their perspective, will be a tricky task, and is something we explore more in Chapter 7. You should definitely enlist the help of national decision makers, and a panel as influential as the Chicago panel on neuroblastoma would be the ideal, although public values and beliefs may make this impossible (see Chapter 8). The situation also reflects what is currently happening with prostate screening.

Chapter 5

Question one

(a) First of all you will make sure you have read any national policy statements, objectives, guidance, etc., and any information about what funding is available and how this is to be obtained. Equipped with this information you can then use the prgramme map (p. 131) as a checklist to draw up some headings about the main tasks. A lot will depend on what is being done nationally or regionally, whether specific organizations have been given responsibility for leading relevant processes, and therefore what you have to do locally. There may be an opportunity to visit somewhere that has already implemented to learn from their experience.

(b) The key people to be members of your Implementation Group are probably as follows, although you will undoubtedly hold some larger meetings and there will be some delegation to more junior staff for regular attendance. More people will be involved in the work of subgroups:

- project manager
- two service user representatives, from local support groups; alternatively you may advertise to find them
- someone from the regional screening centre
- the lead endoscopist from the hospital that will host the screening unit
- a business manager from the same hospital
- whoever will be the pathology lead
- representatives from cancer teams that will receive referrals from the screening unit
- communications lead
- information management and technology representative
- representative from the Regional Quality Assurance Team (if in existence yet)
- a colleague from your finance team, and one from your contracts/commissioning team
- representative from 'primary care' (i.e. the family doctor services).

Question two

(a) Main concerns are:

- The haphazard service provision will be causing confusion and distress for many parents who are unsure as to what tests they need and whether they should pay for private provision.
- The investment of medical and nursing time devoted to Down's screening is more than enough to ensure a high quality service for all, but is inequitably distributed, with some people getting no service and others having investigations that they do not need.

- There is no consistent policy, no consistent training and no consistent quality standards, with the result that some couples are receiving inaccurate and misleading advice and some are receiving tests that are not performed to rigorous standards. At worst this could mean that miscarriage rates from amniocentesis are higher than they should be, and that the risks of performing termination for a baby that is actually normal are higher than they should be. It also means that couples with a Down's baby are likely to go undetected even though they have chosen to participate in screening.

(b) The first step that you need to take is to assemble information about the current provision, and summarize it in a report that includes very clear and explicit explanation of why the current provision is unsatisfactory. This will take some work, and you will need to assemble information about the numbers of couples being screened, the tests being offered, the quality standards being followed, the numbers referred for amniocentesis, and so on. If providers refuse to supply you with information this needs to be made explicit in the report.

You can then use this information to raise awareness about the unsatisfactory position, by sending it as a draft version to all the relevant parties. Use strong wording in the draft—no diplomatic understatement. Make it clear that you are asking for their confirmation of the accuracy of the technical data and that the report is destined for an open meeting of a relevant board. Board meetings are public meetings and are attended by the local press. This may attract people's attention and be sufficient to get them committed to working with you to improve matters.

If despite all this there is still complete refusal to start working on improving matters, then you need to escalate matters by sharing your concerns with regional and national bodies responsible for the quality of antenatal screening, local and national consumer groups and perhaps the media. Once there is sufficient recognition of the problems and of the need for change, then you can work with people to formulate plans for securing a high quality Down's syndrome screening service locally. Producing such plans single-handedly before there is awareness of the problems is usually a waste of time and tends to provoke activity aimed at resisting any change.

Chapter 6

Question one

The objectives, criteria and standards correspond as follows:

A H M

B F N

C I K

D J O

E G L

Question two

It is very unlikely that you will have hit on the same examples as we have, but the process of thinking through the consequences of not meeting standards is a helpful exercise in itself. Here is one example, for each of objectives B–E, of what could go wrong if quality standards are not met. Another aspect of quality assurance that we have not covered in this question is the fact that once you run screening programmes for millions of people and from all walks of life, it is only a matter of time before you encounter people who move, change name, go in and out of prison, have the same name as someone else in their house, and every other eventuality that challenges those delivering screening. The systems have to be able to cope with this.

B. **Timely results.** A woman accepts antenatal screening when she is 12 weeks pregnant, and her screening result shows she is a carrier. She has to wait to receive information about partner testing, and then the father's test result is also delayed by 3 weeks. He proves to be a carrier too, and on prenatal testing the foetus is found to be homozygous. By this stage, the woman is 21 weeks pregnant and the couple now face the prospect of a late termination. They opt for termination, they name the baby and have a burial ceremony. They believe that the delays added significantly to their distress and they have great difficulty coming to terms with their experience.

C. **Expertise in counselling.** A couple has a complex family history and already has a child with severe disabilities. They explain to their midwife that they definitely do not want to go through with the pregnancy if the foetus has a seriously debilitating condition. Their screening result indicates a low risk and the midwife reassures them, wrongly, that this means the foetus is definitely unaffected. Had the midwife been properly trained, then she would have referred them to the genetics service and prenatal diagnosis would have been offered. The baby is born with a serious haemoglobinopathy.

D. **Minimize adverse effects.** A woman accepts screening antenatally and proves to be a carrier for thalassaemia. She confides to the midwife that the true father of the baby is not her husband and, with support from the midwife, the baby's real father is tested. This shows he is also a carrier. Newborn testing reveals that the baby has only inherited one version of the affected gene so the baby does not have thalassaemia and is only a carrier. The mother does not disclose any of this to her husband. Information sent to the family doctor and filed in the mother's record is ambiguous, and says 'mother and father both positive for thalassaemia trait, baby tested heterozygous'. A year later, the married couple come to see the family doctor as they are now expecting a second baby. The doctor asks them what their feelings are about thalassaemia in view of their screening records, and this provokes an uncomfortable silence. The husband asks what the doctor means, and the wife says that there must be some mistake. Subsequently she consults the doctor on her own, explains the full story, and he explains the mistake in the notes. Matters are resolved satisfactorily but a damaging breach of confidentiality could have occurred.

E. **Accurate prenatal diagnosis.** A Cypriot mother accepts antenatal screening for haemoglobinopathy and tests positive as a carrier for β-thalassaemia. There is a history of thalassaemia in her family, and her partner, who is also Cypriot, is tested, and is also a thalassaemia carrier, so they choose to have chorionic villus sampling early in the pregnancy to establish a diagnosis in the baby. The report from the prenatal testing laboratory says that the baby is only a carrier for thalassaemia and the couple feel very relieved. Once the baby is born, it is unwell and tests reveal that the child is in fact homozygous for β-thalassaemia. The consultant explains to the couple that prenatal diagnosis is technically difficult, even in the best units it only achieves a correct result 99 per cent of the time, and several factors can contribute to an inaccurate result. The consultant promises a full case review and to keep them fully informed, but the couple believe that had they been cared for in London this would not have happened. They contact the local newspaper because they are desperate to get improvements in services for haemoglobin disorders. The laboratory is unable to provide the newspaper with any data to show that they are achieving high performance for prenatal diagnosis, so the news coverage is highly damaging and leads to substantial loss of public confidence in the service.

Note: These questions are based on standards developed for the NHS sickle cell and thalassaemia screening programme (NHS Sickle Cell and Thallassaemia Programme 2006) although some aspects have been simplified for these questions. Further information about the programme is available in the National Library for Health Screening Sublibrary (NHS National Library for Health Screening Sublibrary 2006).

Chapter 7

Question one

When you check on the web to find the national policy and evidence, you discover that the UK national screening committee has reviewed the evidence. Their recommendation is that primary prevention of iron deficiency anaemia in infants is very important but that routine screening is not recommended. You discover that similar advice exists in other countries including the USA, that there are very clear guidelines about infant feeding practices to guard against iron deficiency, and that there are limitations to the screening tests used for anaemia.

You therefore conclude that this is an issue that you should be concerned about because the best protection for your local infants is high quality advice and support from your health visitor workforce and others. Provision of screening tests will divert resources, bring little or no extra benefit and will do some harm. If your department sanctions or funds the screening for the few practices that are doing it now, this will appear to endorse the practice, and neighbouring localities will then ask why there is not a district-wide programme. So if you avoid the problem and fail to address the policy issue with the practices that are screening now, you are likely to increase the conflict that will take place later on.

The things you need to do include the following:

* Contact the practices asking for an opportunity to discuss their proposals for a local screening service.

* Talk to the director of the health visiting service, and to colleagues in the health education and health promotion services, to find out exactly what support is provided for parents in these practices concerning infant feeding. You will particularly want to know if there are special resources for the different ethnic minority communities.

* Provide a briefing for those who will be assessing the business case and who will be making decisions about funding, so that they are aware that the screening service is contrary to national policy and that primary prevention is the appropriate strategy.

* Meet with staff from the practices to listen to their concerns, to hear why they wish to perform screening, and to share with them some of your concerns about why screening might not be the best course of action. You will want to explain that their proposal contravenes national recommendations, and you will want to ask how they are gaining informed consent, with particular emphasis on whether they are explaining to parents that screening is against national recommendations, will falsely reassure in some cases where there is anaemia, and will lead to unnecessary investigations in some cases without anaemia.

* Work with the practice staff and others to prepare a strategy for strengthening the primary prevention of infant iron deficiency anaemia in your multicultural populations.

* At all times keep your Director of Public Health, and other relevant colleagues, informed about your actions.

Question two

If at all possible, it is best to rearrange your commitments so that you can go to the studio and be involved in a three-way discussion. If you do not take part at all, the presenter may say 'the local health authority refused to comment'. If you take part only on a phone line, you are at a disadvantage. In the studio, you can establish a rapport with the interviewer and the other interviewee. You have a much better chance of conveying to the listeners the fact that you share the family doctor's concerns about infant anaemia, that prevention work is well under way and that the controversy is just about the tests.

Key soundbites might be:

◆ Infant anaemia is an important problem but the good news is that it is much less common now than it was 30 years ago.

◆ The most important thing is to give babies and toddlers all the nutrients they need in their everyday diet. Breast milk is best, ordinary cows' milk should not be introduced until 12 months as it is too low in iron so use an infant formula milk instead, weaning onto solids at 6 months needs a variety of iron-rich foods. (Make sure to check the most up to date advice before you go on air and if possible get a leaflet or factsheet that listeners can obtain by phoning in to the radio station, or that can be linked to the radio station's webpage.)

◆ Blood testing for all infants is against national recommendations in both the UK and the USA, this is because they can falsely reassure or, conversely, they can lead to unnecessary investigations for babies that do not have anaemia.

◆ Local services provide expert advice and support for all families through the health visiting service, and the health promotion specialist team is working closely with all the ethnic minority communities.

Question three

The first question you have to ask yourself is whether this is your concern, does solving the training funding issue come under the heading of ensuring that a high quality programme is in place? The answer is yes, because sample takers who are not well trained and up to date with the programme and policy will be giving poor advice and support, will be unlikely to follow guidance about frequency, follow-up and failsafe, will not understand their duties in relation to liasing with call/recall staff and laboratory staff, will not know how to get extra help for reaching the hard to reach groups, and they may fail to recognize or act on clinical problems that need referral or treatment. So you do need at least to take an interest in this problem.

The next question to ask yourself is whose direct responsibility is it to solve the problem and what should you do to help.

- The nurse director should actually take responsibility for solving the problem, so it is important to offer support whilst not actually undermining her role or getting left with the responsibility yourself.

- You will need to talk to the nurse director to find out what steps have been taken already, what is happening in other areas and what all the possible funding sources might be.

- Put it as an agenda item for the next meeting of your local co-ordinating group, and keep it on the agenda until the matter is solved.

- If necessary put it in the Annual Report as part of the list of actions to be achieved in the forthcoming year.

- Get directly involved if no progress is being made.

Question four

We do not think that there is a right or wrong answer to this question, and we suspect that most public health practitioners, ourselves included, would do nothing other than keeping the advertisement on file in case anything else happened. Nobody has actually contacted you with concerns about the clinic, and this is probably only one out of numerous small-scale unscientific commercial practices happening in your locality. At most we might pass on the details, together with the results of our web search, to a trusted journalist (if we knew of one) who takes an interest in this type of issue.

If the advertising became more aggressive and overtly misleading claims were being made, or if you became aware of complaints about the service, then it would be appropriate to raise concerns with relevant authorities.

Chapter 8

Question one

(a) Your answer (see p. 221) should say something about natural frequencies being a method of presenting numerical probabilities in a way that people find easy to understand, that uses simple numbers and an explanation that matches how people experience things in life. Gigerenzer actually defines natural frequencies as 'numbers that correspond to the way humans experienced information before the invention of probability theory'. So a statement such as 'if ten people with arthritis like yours take this drug for a year, one person out of the ten is likely to experience an important improvement in their arthritis symptoms'. This is in contrast to a statement such as 'this drug gives a ten per cent improvement in arthritis'—which is ambiguous: it could mean everyone gets a ten per cent improvement, or ten per cent get a benefit, and the benefit could be in symptoms or could be in pathological measures that do not relate to symptoms, and it depends on the person understanding what a percentage is.

(b) Your answer (see p. 223) should say something about framing being the way that numerical data are presented and set in context, and that it has an influence on the way people make decisions consequent on the data. Examples could include the use of relative risk to make an effect seem more significant when the absolute risk change is actually small. For example, if you buy three lottery tickets instead of one you 'treble your chances of winning', and you 'increase your chance of winning by less than one in a million'. The statements are both true but are differently framed.

(c) Your answer (see p. 225) should say something about balance meaning that you apply exactly consistent techniques to the presentation of information for and against. An example might be that when presenting information about harms and benefits, if you present one as national benefit then the other must be too, and if you put one in font size 14 and on the first page of the leaflet then the other must be font size 14 and on the first page too.

Question two

There is always room for disagreement about what is right and wrong in policy making, but here are our answers:

(a) Disagree, all screening does harm, some does good as well.

(b) Disagree, test accuracy does not tell you about the benefits and harms of the programme (see Chapter 4).

(c) Agree, policy makers must always look at whole programme costs, not just the cost of the test. If screening is introduced, resources will be needed for diagnostic services for those with positive screening results, support services (both short term and long term) for parents and infants with positive results, staff training, programme co-ordination, and quality assurance systems.

(d) Disagree, the policy makers have not assembled any evidence about whether any babies benefit from the tests. There needs to be much more information about the purpose of screening, case definitions, interventions and outcomes. There needs to be evidence from trials that measure whether beneficial outcomes can be achieved and how much harm is done.

(e) Disagree, equity in this instance is achieved by protecting all infants from unvalidated potentially harmful interventions. If some laboratories are performing testing that has yet to be evaluated as a screening programme, then the policy makers should recommend that the practice either be stopped, or that the testing is conducted only as part of proper research.

(f) Disagree, input from patients and consumers is necessary but not sufficient for policy; good quality evidence is needed too.

(g) Agree, this is necessary to find what evidence already exists, so that policy can be decided or appropriate research commissioned.

(h) Disagree, this is necessary but not sufficient.

(i) Disagree, policy makers should do their job properly even if they face adversity.

(j) Agree, this will be a harm.

(k) Disagree, these outcomes are inevitable. If there is real benefit then screening may still be the right thing to do, but the harms need to be explained to potential participants and quality standards need to be put in place that keep them to a minimum.

Note: there are similarities between the scenario given in this question, and the much criticized approach to policy making adopted in 2005 by the American College of Medical Genetics (Botkin *et al.* 2006).

Question three

(a) False. Although J.S. Mill was a Utilitarian, he also stated very clearly in *On liberty* that individuals should be free to make their own decisions even if they chose to ignore beneficial interventions (provided it did not harm others).

(b) True.

(c) False. Moral philosophers view this as a supremely difficult question, but it is hard to argue an ethical difference.

(d) False. It is called 'autonomy'

(e) False. This used to be the implicit policy in the past, but since 2001 the explicit policy of the UK National Screening Programmes is that the purpose of information about screening is to ensure that individuals can make an informed choice about whether to participate in screening.

(f) False. It is against the law to discriminate against any individual solely on the grounds of age, but this does not mean that age cut-offs for offering screening are unlawful provided that the policy has been lawfully made, is based on proper and full consideration of evidence and other relevant considerations, and that there is transparency and accountability.

(g) True.

(h) False. Secret decisions are not regarded as fair. The 'veil of ignorance theory' says we should choose rules that create a society we would be comfortable with whatever our place in it. So the ignorance is about imagining you are ignorant as to your position.

(i) True.

Glossary

AABR and AOAE: abbreviations for screening tests used in newborn hearing screening.

Alzheimer's disease: degeneration of the central nervous system associated with age. It is the most common cause of what is commonly called dementia.

Amniocentesis: needle aspiration to remove sample of amniotic fluid for examination. This makes it possible to examine cells from the foetus.

Angiography: an imaging technique used to make arteries visible for X-ray examination. It involves injection of contrast medium via a tube inserted into an artery.

Aortic aneurysm: abnormal dilatation of a segment of the aorta, the main artery leading from the heart.

Audiological assessment: clinical examination of newborn infants identified as having a possible hearing defect.

Bacteruria: the presence of bacteria in the urine.

Bias: a systematic error resulting from prejudice.

Bimodal: when the values of a variable in a population are distributed in such a way that it appears that there are two subgroups in the population, namely two peaks in the frequency distribution curve.

Biopsy: a sample of tissue taken for examination.

Birth cohort: group of people born in a specified time interval.

Blinded ascertainment: a technique for avoiding bias; the person who is doing the assessment does not know, for example, the previous professional's assessment, or whether the subject being assessed has received intervention or placebo.

Bloodspot test: term used to describe the blood tests offered routinely to newborn infants. The sample is obtained by pricking the baby's heel.

Breast self-examination: a technique in which a woman systematically examines her breasts for lumps.

Britain/British: strictly speaking Britain is the large island comprising England, Wales and Scotland, but it is often used loosely to mean the United Kingdom of Great Britain and Northern Island. The British Isles refers to all the islands, including all of Ireland.

BSE: see breast self-examination.

Case–control study: a research method in which, for each person with the condition being studied (a case), another person as like the person with the disease as possible except for the absence of disease (a control) is identified for long-term follow-up or for enquiry into lifestyle or environment. The study analyses differences between the cases and controls.

Case definition: specific definition of what constitutes a case.

Case-finding: this is difficult to define as it tends to be used rather vaguely. It can mean finding cases in known high risk individuals.

Cervical carcinoma *in situ*: term used in the early days of cervical screening to describe tissue change in the cervix, now replaced by the term cervical intraepithelial neoplasia.

Cervix cancer: cancer of the neck of the womb—the 'cervix uteri'.

Cervical intraepithelial neoplasia: pathologically defined abnormal appearance in cervical biopsy, it has grades of severity, with grade three being the worst.

Cervical screening test: a sample of cells from the cervix is obtained during vaginal examination, and is sent to a laboratory where the cells are examined using a high power microscope. The test may be a 'smear' where the sample is spread on a glass slide, or a 'liquid-based' sample where cells are placed in liquid.

Chlamydia: a unicellular organism that is commonly found in men and women. Infection with chlamydia can lead to fertility problems in women.

Chromosome: the long sequence of nucleic acid in the nucleus of the cell. It contains the genes.

Clinically diagnosed: diagnosed because of symptoms or signs.

Cochlear implant: implantation of a device to treat deafness. It reproduces the functions of the inner ear or cochlea.

The Cochrane Collaboration: an international collaboration devoted to the preparation and maintenance of systematic reviews.

Colonoscopy: the inspection of the interior of the colon with a flexible endoscope.

Colposcopy: the direct inspection of the cervix of the uterus using a colposcope which gives a magnified view.

Co-morbidity: the presence of two or more conditions.

Complex genetic disorder: disorder contributed to by the combined effect of several or even many risk variants of genes.

Computerized tomography or CT scan: an X-ray image of a section or multiple sections of the body.

Conductive hearing loss: one of the common causes of deafness, entailing defective transmission of sound through the ear.

Cone biopsy: the excision of a cone of tissue from the cervix of the uterus.

Confidence intervals: statistical limits placed on either side of the research result to indicate the confidence that the research worker has that their results, based on a sample of the whole population, represent the true result if the whole population were measured, the true results for the whole population being, in the confident view of the researcher, at some point in the range of values between these limits.

Confounders: when two groups are being compared which differ with respect to one variable, other variables may be present which make it impossible to ascribe sole responsibility for the cause of a disease to the variable being considered. These other variables are known as confounders.

Congenital hypothyroidism: a condition in which the thyroid gland of the baby does not function properly. If not detected, this can lead to impairment in intellectual development.

Cut-off: an arbitrary point separating results that are deemed positive from those that are deemed negative.

Cytology: the examination of cells using a microscope.

Cytoscreener: someone who examines cells microscopically, for example in cervical screening.

Cystic fibrosis: a genetic disorder in which secretions are of a higher than average viscosity, leading to infection. The lungs are particularly prone to infection.

DCIS: see ductal carcinoma *in situ*.

Decision aid: a tool that helps either a patient or clinician reach a decision. It helps set out likely outcomes of alternative courses of action.

Deep vein thrombosis: the blockage by a blood clot of a vein in a muscle of the limb.

Demonstration project: a project in which a new service is delivered in one population, offering professionals who work in other parts of the health service the opportunity of observing how the service is delivered.

Diabetes mellitus: a disorder characterized by high levels of sugar in the bloodstream and other metabolic problems.

Diabetic retinopathy: damage to the retina resulting from diabetes.

Diagnostic test: a test that aims to give a definitive answer about diagnosis. Screening tests are not usually diagnostic.

Dipstick test: a test in which a small plastic strip with chemicals laid on to it is dipped into the urine. Colour change indicates the result.

Distraction test: a test of hearing in which the tester tries to observe the baby's reaction to a sound stimulus while attempting to focus the baby's attention elsewhere.

DNA (deoxyribonucleic acid): the molecule from which genes are made.

Down's syndrome (sometimes known as trisomy 21): a syndrome resulting from having three rather than two chromosomes number 21. Affected individuals may have intellectual impairment and may have heart defects and other problems.

Dual-energy X-ray (DXA) absorption scan: a scan using low dose X-rays that gives a measure of bone density.

Ductal carcinoma *in situ*: a borderline pathological condition found in breast tissue. It was not diagnosed before screening began.

DXA scan: see dual-energy X-ray scan.

Electrocardiogram: electrical tracing of the heart's activity.

Elective: planned as opposed to emergency.

Embryo: term used to describe the developing human young during the first 7–9 weeks from fertilization, during which time the major organs are formed.

Endoscopy: the visual examination of some interior part of the body, for example the colon or stomach, using a fibreoptic tube.

Enzyme: a chemical that accelerates the interaction of two other chemicals.

Epidemiological: research method that studies populations rather than individuals.

Evidence-based: decision making that is based on best current knowledge derived from research.

Exercise electrocardiogram: electrical tracing of the heart's activity recorded whilst the subject exercises on a treadmill.

Faecal occult blood: blood that is present in the faeces but is not obvious and has to be detected by biochemical reaction.

Failsafe system: a back-up mechanism that ensures that if some-thing goes wrong in a system, then action ensues to ensure a safe outcome. In screening programmes, failsafe is designed to ensure that individuals are followed-up appropriately.

False-negative result: a negative test result in a person who does have the condition being tested for.

False-positive result: a positive test result in a person who does not have the condition being tested for.

Familial: occurring more often in a family than would be expected by chance. Familial diseases may be either genetic or environmental.

Fibreoptic: a type of flexible endoscope.

Foetus: the developing human young from about 9 weeks after fertilization until birth.

Genetic: influenced by genes.

Genetic carrier: someone who has a genetic mutation but does not develop a disease as a result of it.

Genetic screening: a term that is widely used but has no specific meaning and should not be used.

Genetic test: a test to detect a genetic mutation.

Genotype: a description of an individual's genetic status.

Glaucoma: a disorder of the eye characterized by raised pressure within the eyeball.

Haematological: relating to blood.

Heaf test: test for tuberculosis.

Health maintenance organization: a health insurance scheme which covers all aspects of the care of enrolled people.

Health visitor: public health nurse.

Healthy screenee effect: term used to describe the fact that people who come for screening tend to be healthier than those who do not. This makes it impossible to know (without a proper control group) whether better outcomes in screened individuals are caused by the screening, or whether they are the result you would expect anyway when observing a self-selected group of healthier people.

Heelprick test: obtaining a spot of blood from the newborn infant by heelprick.

Histology: microscopic examination of human tissue.

HIV: human immunodeficiency virus.

Huntington's disease: a serious neurological disease caused by the inheritance of a certain genetic mutation. Onset is usually in adulthood.

Hypertension: synonym for high blood pressure.

Hysterectomy: operation to remove the uterus.

Implantation: placing of fertilized eggs in the uterus.

Incidence: number of new cases occurring within a population within a specified time period, usually a year.

Inconsequential disease: detectable pathological change or risk markers that would never lead to clinical disease in the persons lifetime. Also known as latent disease or pseudodisease.

Interval cancer: cancer arising between two screening tests.

***In vitro* fertilization (IVF)**: artificial insemination of an ovum in the laboratory.

Iron deficiency anaemia: reduced level of haemoglobin resulting either from deficient iron intake or, more usually, from excessive blood loss.

Kaiser Permanente: a health insurance plan available to residents of San Francisco.

Karyotype: a description of an individual with regard to the number of chromosomes they have.

Laparoscopic: direct visualisation of a human cavity such as the abdomen.

Laser treatment: treatment with a focused source of heat.

Latent disease: see inconsequential disease.

Lead time effect: survival time for people with screen-detected disease appears longer because you start the clock sooner.

Length time effect: phenomenon whereby screening appears effective because screening is best at picking up long-lasting non-progressive or slowly progressive pathological conditions. This pulls good prognosis cases into your group of screen-detected cases, and leaves out the poor prognosis rapidly progressive cases that screening has little chance of detecting. This means that the outcome in a group of screen-detected cases is automatically better than the outcome in a group of clinically diagnosed cases even if screening makes no difference to outcome.

Liquid-based cytology: a type of cervical screening test in which the cell sample is put into liquid, and prepared in the laboratory ready for visual examination.

Live blood analysis: a test of no scientific validity practised by quacks.

Loop excision: the removal of a part of the uterine cervix using a loop of heated wire.

Magnetic resonance imaging (MRI): a type of imaging that produces images of much higher detail within soft tissues than is possible by X-ray.

Mammography: imaging of the breast.

Mastectomy: removal of the breast.

Medical Officer of Health: a post created in 1857 and abolished in 1974 where a public health doctor is responsible for a defined population within the UK.

Mendelian inheritance: derived from the work of Mendel who first described the pattern of dominant inheritance where the inheritance of a single genetic mutation resulted in some obvious feature in the offspring.

Metabolite: a substance produced by the breakdown of large complex chemicals in the body.

Microscopic haematuria: blood in the urine detected only by microscopic examination of the urine and not by the naked eye.

Modelling: a technique by which the costs, risks and benefits of an intervention or service can be statistically predicted.

Morbidity: a synonym for illness.

Multiphasic examination: multiple tests performed automatically.

Mutation: a change in a gene, which may or may not lead to a disease.

Natural history: what would happen to the condition in that individual in the absence of any intervention.

Negative predictive value: the probability that an individual does not have the condition being tested for, given that the result is negative.

Opportunistic screening: the use of contact with a person initiated because that person has symptoms, to offer a screening test.

Opportunity cost: the opportunity cost of an innovation is measured by the services that could be funded by the amount of resources for that innovation if a decision were made to invest in another service.

Overdetection: see overdiagnosis.

Overdiagnosis: the phenomenon whereby screening diagnoses cases that would never have been clinically manifest in the person's lifetime.

Overinvestigation: carrying out medical diagnostic investigations in low risk individuals.

Overtreatment: the phenomenon whereby screening leads to treatment of cases that would never have been clinically manifest in the person's lifetime.

Papanicolou: Greek doctor credited with inventing the cervical screening test.

Pathological change: detectable change away from what is considered normal.

Peer-reviewed: a research proposal or journal article reviewed by other scientists.

Periodic examination: an examination that takes place at fixed periods of time.

Phenistix: a type of biochemical test.

Phenotype: the physical characteristics of an individual arising from a combination of genetic and environmental influences, as opposed to a genotype which is the genetic status of the individual.

Phenylalanine: an amino acid.

Phenylketonuria (PKU): an inherited disease characterized by deficient ability to process phenylalanine.

Pilot project: when a new service is introduced it is often used in one part of the country to identify areas of potential difficulty and to develop resources for nationwide implementation.

Polyp: a raised piece of tissue, for example in the lining of the bowel.

Popularity paradox: because of overdiagnosis and overtreatment, far more people believe they have derived benefit from screening than is actually the case.

Positive predictive value: the probability that an individual has the condition being tested for, given that the result is positive.

Post-test probability: the probability that an individual has a disease if they have a positive test result.

Pre-cancer: a misleading term used to describe cells and tissues that look like cancer cells but are not behaving like cancer cells. These abnormal-looking cells are a very common phenomenon.

Preimplantation genetic testing: testing for mutations in fertilized eggs.

Pre-test probability: the probability that an individual has a disease before they have a test.

Prevalence: the number of cases of a condition in the population at any point in time.

Prognosis: the likely clinical outcome in an individual diagnosed with a condition.

Prostate-specific antigen test (PSA): measurement of a protein in the blood which indicates the size of the prostate.

Pseudodisease: see inconsequential disease.

Pulmonary embolism: a blood clot lodged in the pulmonary artery.

Pulmonary tuberculosis: tuberculosis affecting the lungs.

Quality assurance processes: techniques for minimizing error and improving performance against explicit standards.

Randomized controlled trial: a research method to assess the effectiveness of a treatment or service. Subjects are assigned randomly either to receive an intervention or to be in the control group.

Receiver operator characteristic curve: a way of illustrating, on one graph, and for one test, the sensitivity and specificity achieved at any cut-off level and the trade-off between them.

Relative risk: the risk that an individual will develop a condition compared with the general risk in the population.

Rhesus haemolytic disease: disease of the newborn in which red blood cells are destroyed because of incompatibility between the infant's blood cells and antibodies to the blood cells of the mother.

ROC curve: see receiver operator characteristic curve.

Screening programme: whole system of activities needed to deliver high quality screening.

Screening test: a test or inquiry used on people who do not have or have not recognized the signs or symptoms of the condition being tested for. It divides people into low and higher risk groups.

Selection bias: a reason for error in a research project because of the tendency of individuals conducting research to select one group or another preferentially.

Sensitivity: ability of a test to correctly identify cases as positive.

Sensori-neural hearing loss: deafness due to disorders of the nerves or brain.

Sieve: a useful word to describe the screening phase in a screening programme.

Sickle cell disorders: inherited conditions involving disorders of the red blood cells.

Signs and symptoms: changes in the individual detected by the patient or clinician; symptoms are what the patient feels is wrong with them, signs are physically observable phenomena.

Single gene disorder: diseases, usually rare, caused by a variation (a mutation) in a single gene. Inheritance follows the traditional 'Mendelian' pattern. Examples are Huntington's disease and Duchenne muscular dystrophy.

Sort: a useful word to describe the diagnostic phase in a screening programme.

Specificity: ability of a test correctly to identify non-cases as negative.

Surveillance: hard to define, but generally used to mean keeping an eye on things.

Tandem mass spectrometry: a technique for measuring the levels of multiple chemicals in the blood.

Thalassaemia: inherited disorder of the red blood cells.

Time trend analysis: measurement of changes over a long period of time.

Tumour markers: proteins or other detectable substances that may indicate the presence of a tumour in the body.

Ultrasound: the use of sound waves to detect solid objects, for example tumours in the liver.

Unimodal: the distribution of a variable in the population showing only one peak in frequency.

References

Chapter 1

Anderson, C.M. (1997) *Lawyers, ethicists, and consumers want greater honesty about cervical screening*, Manchester: Multi-disciplinary Workshop, Manchester Business School.

Anderson, C.M. and Thornton, J.G. (1994) Screening for cervical cancer. Graphs may mislead. *British Medical Journal* 309, 953–954.

Anderson, O.W. and Rosen, G. (1960) An examination of the concept of preventive medicine. *Health Information Research Foundation Series* 12, 17–18.

Anonymous (1985) Cancer of the cervix: death by incompetence. *Lancet* 2, 363–364.

Boyes, D.A., Morrison, B., Knox, E.G., Draper, G.J. and Miller, A.B. (1982) A cohort study of cervical cancer screening in British Columbia. *Clinical and Investigative Medicine* 5, 1–29.

Canadian Task Force on the Periodic Health Examination (1979) The periodic health examination. *Canadian Medical Association Journal* 121, 1193–1254.

Childers, E. (1903) *The riddle of the sands*. London: Penguin Books.

Cochrane, A. (1971) *Effectiveness and efficiency. Random reflections on health services*. Cambridge: Cambridge University Press.

Cochrane, A. (1976) Some reflections. In: Nuffield Provincial Hospitals Trust, ed. *A question of quality? Roads to assurance in medical care*. Oxford: Oxford University Press.

Collen, M.F. (1974) Multiphasic testing as a triage to medical care. In: Ingelfinger, F.J., ed. *Controversy in internal medicine*, Vol. 2. Philadelphia: W.B. Saunders, pp. 85–91.

Commission on Chronic Illness (1957) *Chronic illness in the United States*, Vol. 1. Cambridge MA: Harvard University Press.

Cook, C. (2004) Oral history—Walter Holland. *Journal of Public Health* 26, 121–129.

Department of Health and Social Security (1988) *Health Services Management cervical cancer screening*. HC(88)1. London: DHSS.

Dobell, H. (1861) *Lectures on the germs and vestiges of disease, and on the prevention of the invasion and fatality of disease by periodical examinations*. London: Churchill, pp. 142–146.

Evans, N.J.B. (1995) *Review of the Department of Health's arrangements for obtaining external medical and scientific advice*. London: Department of Health.

Frame, P.S. (1986) A critical review of adult health maintenance. Part 1. Prevention of atherosclerotic diseases. *Journal of Family Practice* 22, 341–346.

Frame, P.S. (1986) A critical review of adult health maintenance. Part 2. Prevention of infectious diseases. *Journal of Family Practice* 22, 417–422.

Frame, P.S. (1986) A critical review of adult health maintenance. Part 3. Prevention of cancer. *Journal of Family Practice* 22, 511–520.

Frame, P.S. and Carlson, S.J. (1975a) A critical review of periodic health screening using specific screening criteria. Part 1: selected diseases of respiratory, cardiovascular, and central nervous systems. *Journal of Family Practice* 2, 29–36.

Frame, P.S. and Carlson, S.J. (1975b) A critical review of periodic health screening using specific screening criteria. Part 2: Selected endocrine, metabolic and gastrointestinal diseases. *Journal of Family Practice* 2, 123–129.

Frame, P.S. and Carlson, S.J. (1975c) A critical review of periodic health screening using specific screening criteria. 3. Selected diseases of the genitourinary system. *Journal of Family Practice* 2, 189–194.

Friedman, G.D., Collen, M.F. and Fireman, B.H. (1986) Multiphasic health checkup evaluation: a 16-year follow-up. *Journal of Chronic Diseases* 39, 453–463.

Gellner, E. (1992) *Postmodernism, reason, and religion.* Oxford: Oxford University Press.

Gould, G.M. (1900) A system of personal biological examinations the condition of adequate medical and scientific conduct of life. *Journal of the American Medical Association* 134–137.

Han, P.K. (1997) Historical changes in the objectives of the periodic health examination. *Annals of Internal Medicine* 127, 910–917.

Holland, W.W. (1974) Taking stock. *Lancet* 2, 1494–1497.

Holland, W.W. and Stewart, S. (2005) *Screening in disease prevention, what works?* Oxford: The Nuffield Trust.

Inter-Departmental Committee on Physical Degeneration (1904) Parliamentary Papers.

Knox, E.G. (1982) Cancer of the uterine cervix. In: Magnus, K., ed. *Trends in cancer incidence.* Washington: Hemisphere.

Knox, E.G. (1976) Ages and frequencies for cervical cancer screening. *British Journal of Cancer* 34, 444–452.

Macgregor, J.E., Campbell, M.K., Mann, E.M. and Swanson, K.Y. (1994) Screening for cervical intraepithelial neoplasia in north east Scotland shows fall in incidence and mortality from invasive cancer with concomitant rise in preinvasive disease. *British Medical Journal* 308, 1407–1411.

Martin, J. (2006) *The Meaning of the 21st Century.* Transworld Publishers. London.

McCormick, J.S. (1989) Cervical smears: a questionable practice? *Lancet* 2, 207–209.

McKeown, T. (1968) Validation of screening procedures. In: Nuffield Provincial Hospitals Trust, ed. *Screening in medical care: reviewing the evidence. A collection of essays.* London: Nuffield Provincial Hospitals Trust, pp. 1–13.

McKeown, T. (1976) *Role of medicine: dream mirage or nemesis?* London: Nuffield Provincial Hospitals Trust.

Murphy, M.F., Campbell, M.J. and Goldblatt, P.O. (1988) Twenty years' screening for cancer of the uterine cervix in Great Britain, 1964–84: further evidence for its ineffectiveness. *Journal of Epidemiology and Community Health* 42, 49–53.

National Audit Office (1992) *Report by the Comptroller and Auditor General, cervical and breast screening in England.* 236. London: Her Majesty's Stationery Office.

NHS Cervical Screening programme (2001) *Cervical screening—an informed choice.* NHS Cervical Screening Programme.

NHS Cancer Screening Programmes (2006) NHS Cancer Screening Programmes Website. www.cancerscreening.nhs.uk Sheffield [accessed June 2006].

Nuffield Provincial Hospitals Trust (1968) *Screening in medical care: reviewing the evidence. A collection of essays.* London: Oxford University Press.

Quinn, M., Babb, P., Jones, J. and Allen, E. (1999) Effect of screening on incidence of and mortality from cancer of cervix in England: evaluation based on routinely collected statistics. *British Medical Journal* 318, 904–908.

Raffle, A.E., Alden, B. and Mackenzie, E.F. (1995) Detection rates for abnormal cervical smears: what are we screening for? *Lancet* 345, 1469–1473.

Raffle, A.E., Alden, B., Quinn, M., Babb, P.J. and Brett, M.T. (2003) Outcomes of screening to prevent cancer: analysis of cumulative incidence of cervical abnormality and modelling of cases and deaths prevented. *British Medical Journal* 326, 901.

Rosen, G. (1975) *Preventive medicine in the United States, 1900–1975: trends and interpretations.* New York: Science History.

Sasamori, N. (1982) The present condition of the human dry dock in Japan and its outlook for the future. *Japan Hospitals* 1, 49–55.

Sasieni, P. and Adams, J. (1999) Effect of screening on cervical cancer mortality in England and Wales: analysis of trends with an age period cohort model. *British Medical Journal* 318, 1244–1245.

Sasieni, P., Cuzick, J. and Farmery, E. (1995) Accelerated decline in cervical cancer mortality in England and Wales. *Lancet* 346, 1566–1567.

Scottish Office (1993) *Report of the inquiry into cervical cytopathology at Inverclyde Royal Hospital, Greenock.* Edinburgh: HMSO.

Sharp, F., Duncan, I.D., Evans, D.M.D., *et al.* (1987) *Report of the Intercollegiate Working Party on Cervical Cytology Screening.* London: Royal College of Obstetricians and Gynaecologists.

Skrabanek, P. (1988) Cervical cancer screening: the time for reappraisal. *Canadian Journal of Public Health* 79, 86–89.

Slater, D. (1998) The cervical screening muddle. *Lancet* 351, 1130.

Smith, F.B. (1979) *The people's health 1830 to 1910.* London: Croom Helm.

South-East London Screening Study Group (1977) A controlled trial of multi-phasic screening in middle-age: results of the South-East London Screening Study. The South-East London Screening Study Group. *International Journal of Epidemiology* 6, 357–363.

Thorner, R.R.Q. (1961) *Principles and procedures in the evaluation of screening for disease.* United States Department of Health.

US Preventive Services Task Force (1989) *Guide to clinical preventive services: an assessment of the effectiveness of 169 interventions; report of the US Preventive Services Task Force.* Baltimore: Williams and Wilkins.

Wells, W. (1997) *Review of cervical screening services at Kent and Canterbury Hospitals NHS Trust.* London: NHS Executive South Thames.

Wilson, J.M.G. and Jungner, G. (1968) *The principles and practice of screening for disease.* Public Health Papers no. 34. Geneva: World Health Organization.

Chapter 2

Bessman, S.P. (1966) Legislation and advances in medical knowledge—acceleration or inhibition? *Journal of Pediatrics* 69, 334–338.

Commission on Chronic Illness (1957) *Chronic illness in the United States*, Vol. 1. Cambridge, MA: Harvard University Press.

Department of Health (2006) Department of Health Publications and Statistics website. www.dh.gov.uk/PublicationsAndStatistics/fs/en [accessed June 2006].

Ferrer, H.P. (1968) Screening for health, theory and practice. London: Butterworths.

Gibbons, R.J., Balady, G.J., Bricker, J.T., *et al.* (2002) CC/AHA 2002 guideline update for exercise testing: summary article: a report of the American College of Cardiology/American Heart Association Task Force on Practice Guidelines (Committee to Update the 1997 Exercise Testing Guidelines). *Circulation* 106, 1883–1892.

Holland, W.W. and Stewart, S. (2005) *Screening in disease prevention. What works?* Oxford: Radcliffe Publishing.

Holtzman, N.A. and Watson, M.S. (1999) Promoting safe and effective genetic testing in the United States. Final report of the Task Force on Genetic Testing. *Journal of Child and Family Nursing* 2, 388–390.

Kenny, A. (2005) *Wittgenstein.* Oxford: Blackwell.

Liddell, M.B., Lovestone, S. and Owen, M.J. (2001) Genetic risk of Alzheimer's disease: advising relatives. *British Journal of Psychiatry* 178, 7–11.

McKeown, T. (1968) Validation of screening procedures. In: Nuffield Provincial Hospitals Trust, ed. *Screening in medical care: reviewing the evidence. A collection of essays.* London: Oxford University Press, pp. 1–13.

Ministry of Health (1963) *Letter from the Chief Medical Officer 9/63.* 4 July 1963.

National Institutes of Health Gene Tests database. www.geneclinics.org [accessed 1 July 2006].

NHS National Library for Health Screening Specialist Sublibrary. www.library.nhs.uk/screening/ [accessed July 2006].

Sanderson, S., Green, A., Preece, M. and Burton, H. (2006) The frequency of inherited metabolic disorders in the West Midlands, United Kingdom. *Archives of Disease in Childhood* 91, 896–899.

UK National Screening Committee NHS Screening website. www.screening.nhs.uk/home.htm [accessed 1 July 2006].

UK National Screening Committee (2000) *Second Report of the UK National Screening Committee.* Departments of Health for England, Scotland, Northern Ireland and Wales.

Wald, N.J. (1994) Guidance on terminology. *Journal of Medical Screening* 1, 76.

Wald, N.J. and Leck, I. (2000) *Antenatal and neonatal screening.* Oxford: Oxford University Press.

Wilson, J.M.G. (1968) Evaluation of prescriptive screening for phenylketonuria. In: Nuffield Provincial Hospitals Trust, ed. *Screening in medical care: reviewing the evidence. A collection of essays.* London: Oxford University Press.

Chapter 3

Barratt, A., Irwig, L., Glasziou, P., *et al.* (1999) Users' guides to the medical literature: XVII. How to use guidelines and recommendations about screening. Evidence-based Medicine Working Group. *Journal of the American Medical Association* 281, 2029–2034.

Baum, M. (2006) Ramifications of screening for breast cancer: consent for screening. *British Medical Journal* 332, 728.

Black, W.C., Nease, R.F., Jr and Tosteson, A.N. (1995) Perceptions of breast cancer risk and screening effectiveness in women younger than 50 years of age. *Journal of the National Cancer Institute* 87, pp. 720–731.

Christiansen, C.L., Wang, F., Barton, M.B., Kreuter, W., Elmore, J.G., Gelfand, A.E. and Fletcher, S.W. (2000) Predicting the cumulative risk of false-positive mammograms. *Journal of the National Cancer Institute* 92, 1657–1666.

Elmore, J.G., Nakano, C.Y., Koepsell, T.D., Desnick, L.M., D'Orsi, C.J. and Ransohoff, D.F. (2003) International variation in screening mammography interpretations in community-based programs. *Journal of the National Cancer Institute* 95, 1384–1393.

Ernster, V.L., Barclay, J., Kerlikowske, K., Grady, D. and Henderson, C. (1996) Incidence of and treatment for ductal carcinoma in situ of the breast. *Journal of the American Medical Association* 275, 913–918.

Gøtzsche, P. (1997) Screening for colorectal cancer. *Lancet* 349, 356.

Gøtzsche, P.C. (2006) Ramifications of screening for breast cancer: overdiagnosis in the Malmö trial was considerably underestimated. *British Medical Journal* 332, 727.

Gøtzsche, P.C. and Nielsen, M. (2006) Screening for breast cancer with mammography. Cochrane Database of Systematic Reviews Art No CD00187 [Issue 4], DOI: 10.1002/14651858.CD001877.pub2. Wiley.

Hardcastle, J.D., Chamberlain, J.O., Robinson, M.H., *et al.* (1996) Randomised controlled trial of faecal-occult-blood screening for colorectal cancer. *Lancet* 348, 1472–1477.

Irwig, L., Houssami, N., Armstrong, B. and Glasziou, P. (2006) Evaluating new screening tests for breast cancer. *British Medical Journal* 332, 678–679.

Johnson, C. (2004) Cancer from the patient's perspective. Speech to Avon Somerset and Wiltshire Cancer Services Annual Conference.

Kronborg, O., Fenger, C., Olsen, J., Jorgensen, O.D. and Sondergaard, O. (1996) Randomised study of screening for colorectal cancer with faecal-occult-blood test. *Lancet* 348, 1467–1471.

Möller, H. and Davies, E. (2006) Over-diagnosis in breast cancer screening. *British Medical Journal* 332, 691–692.

Möller, B., Weedon-Fekjaer, H., Hakulinen, T., Tryggvadottir, L., Storm, H.H., Talback, M. and Haldorsen, T. (2005) The influence of mammographic screening on national trends in breast cancer incidence. *European Journal of Cancer Prevention* 14, 117–128.

National Screening Committee (2003) *Antenatal screening for Down's syndrome—Policy and quality issues.* National Screening Committee.

NHS Breast Screening Programme (2005) *Quality assurance guidelines for breast cancer screening.* Radiology Publication number 59.

Nielsen, M. (1989) Autopsy studies of the occurrence of cancerous, atypical and benign epithelial lesions in the female breast. *APMIS Supplement* 10, 1–56.

Raffle, A.E., Alden, B., Quinn, M., Babb, P.J. and Brett, M.T. (2003) Outcomes of screening to prevent cancer: analysis of cumulative incidence of cervical abnormality and modelling of cases and deaths prevented. *British Medical Journal* 326, 901.

Schmidt, J.G. (1990) The epidemiology of mass breast cancer screening —a plea for a valid measure of benefit. *Journal of Clinical Epidemiology* 43, 215–225.

Scholefield, J.H., Moss, S., Sufi, F., Mangham, C.M. and Hardcastle, J.D. (2002) Effect of faecal occult blood screening on mortality from colorectal cancer: results from a randomised controlled trial. *Gut* 50, 840–844.

Smith-Bindman, R., Chu, P.W., Miglioretti, D.L., *et al.* (2003) Comparison of screening mammography in the United States and the United Kingdom. *Journal of the American Medical Association* 290, pp. 2129–2137.

Thornton, H. (1999) Evidence-based information. *Lancet* 353, 2249.

Thornton, H. (2006) Ramifications of screening for breast cancer: more debate and better information still needed. *British Medical Journal* 332, 728.

UK CRC Screening Pilot Evaluation Team (2003) *Evaluation of the UK Colorectal Cancer Screening Pilot.* Edinburgh: University of Edinburgh.

Ward, D. (1996) Catherine; living with pain. In: *One in 10; women living with breast cancer*. St Leonards NSW Australia: Allen and Unwin, pp. 102–110.

Welch, H.G. (2004) *Should I be tested for cancer? Maybe not and here's why.* Los Angeles: University of California Press.

Welch, H.G. and Black, W.C. (1997) Using autopsy series to estimate the disease 'reservoir' for ductal carcinoma in situ of the breast: how much more breast cancer can we find? *Annals of Internal Medicine* 127, 1023–1028.

Welch, H.G., Schwartz, L.M. and Woloshin, S. (2006) Ramifications of screening for breast cancer: 1 in 4 cancers detected by mammography are pseudocancers. *British Medical Journal* 332, 727.

Zackrisson, S., Andersson, I., Janzon, L., Manjer, J. and Garne, J.P. (2006) Rate of over-diagnosis of breast cancer 15 years after end of Malmo mammographic screening trial: follow-up study, *British Medical Journal* 332, 689–692.

Zahl, P.H. and Maehlen, J. (2006) Ramifications of screening for breast cancer: definition of overdiagnosis is confusing in follow-up of Malmö trial. *British Medical Journal* 332, 727–728.

Zahl, P.H., Strand, B.H. and Maehlen, J. (2004) Incidence of breast cancer in Norway and Sweden during introduction of nationwide screening: prospective cohort study. *British Medical Journal* 328, 921–924.

Chapter 4

Alexander, F.E. and Prescott, R.J. (1999) Reply to Labrie *et al.* Results of the mortality analysis of the Quebec randomized controlled trial (RCT). *Prostate* 40, 135–137.

Barratt, A.L. and Coates, A.S. 2004) Screening decreases prostate cancer death: first analysis of the 1988 Quebec Prospective Randomized Controlled Trial. *Medical Journal of Australia* 181, 213–214.

Bell, R., Petticrew, M., Luengo, S. and Sheldon, T.A. (1998) Screening for ovarian cancer: a systematic review. *Health Technology Assessment* 2, 1–84.

Bhopal, R. (2002) *Concepts of epidemiology. An integrated introduction to the ideas, theories, principles and methods of epidemiology.* Oxford: Oxford University Press.

Boer, R. and Schroder, F.H. (1999) Quebec randomized controlled trial on prostate cancer screening shows no evidence for mortality reduction. *Prostate* 40, 130–134.

Botkin, J.R., Clayton, E.W., Fost, N.C., *et al.* (2006) Newborn screening technology: proceed with caution. *Pediatrics* 117, 1793–1799.

Craft, A.W., Parker, L., Dale, G., *et al.* (1992) A pilot study of screening for neuroblastoma in the north of England. *American Journal of Pediatric Hematology and Oncology* 14, 337–341.

Cronin, K.A., Weed, D.L., Connor, R.J. and Prorok, P.C. (1998) Case–control studies of cancer screening: theory and practice. *Journal of the National Cancer Institute* 90, 498–504.

Elwood, M. (2004) A misleading paper on prostate cancer screening. *Prostate* 61, 372–374.

Elwyn, G., O'Connor, A., Stacey, D., *et al.* (2006) Developing a quality criteria framework for patient decision aids: online international Delphi consensus process. *British Medical Journal* 333, 417.

Family Heart Study Group (1994) Randomised controlled trial evaluating cardiovascular screening and intervention in general practice: principal results of British family heart study. *British Medical Journal* 308, 313–320.

Gibbons, R.J., Balady, G.J., Bricker, J.T., *et al.* (2002) ACC/AHA 2002 guideline update for exercise testing: summary article: a report of the American College of Cardiology/American Heart Association Task Force on Practice Guidelines (Committee to Update the 1997 Exercise Testing Guidelines). *Circulation* 106, 1883–1892.

Gigerenzer, G. (2002) *Reckoning with risk*. London: Penguin.

Hardcastle, J.D., Chamberlain, J.O., Robinson, M.H., *et al.* (1996) Randomised controlled trial of faecal-occult-blood screening for colorectal cancer. *Lancet* 348, 1472–1477.

Kronborg, O., Fenger, C., Olsen, J., Jorgensen, O.D. and Sondergaard, O. (1996) Randomised study of screening for colorectal cancer with faecal-occult-blood test. *Lancet* 348, 1467–1471.

Laara, E., Day, N.E. and Hakama, M. (1987) Trends in mortality from cervical cancer in the Nordic countries: association with organised screening programmes. *Lancet* 1, 1247–1249.

Labrie, F., Candas, B., Dupont, A., *et al.* (1999) Screening decreases prostate cancer death: first analysis of the 1988 Quebec prospective randomized controlled trial. *Prostate* 38, 83–91.

Labrie, F., Candas, B., Cusan, L., *et al.* (2004) Screening decreases prostate cancer mortality: 11-year follow-up of the 1988 Quebec prospective randomized controlled trial. *Prostate* 59, 311–318.

Levi, F., Lucchini, F., Negri, E., Franceschi, S. and la Vecchia, C. (2000) Cervical cancer mortality in young women in Europe: patterns and trends. *European Journal of Cancer* 36, 2266–2271.

Locker, A.P., Caseldine, J., Mitchell, A.K., Blamey, R.W., Roebuck, E.J. and Elston, C.W. (1989) Results from a seven-year programme of breast self-examination in 89,010 women. *British Journal of Cancer* 60, 401–405.

Martyn, C. (1999) Bookcase. *British Medical Journal* 318, 1771.

Moss, S.M. (1991) Case–control studies of screening. *International Journal of Epidemiology* 20, 1–6.

Murphy, S.B., Cohn, S.L., Craft, A.W., *et al.* (1991) Do children benefit from mass screening for neuroblastoma? Consensus Statement from the American Cancer Society Workshop on Neuroblastoma Screening. *Lancet* 337, 344–346.

National Institute for Clinical Excellence (2003) *Guidance on the use of liquid-based cytology for cervical screening. Technology Appraisal 69.* London: NHS.

National Screening Committee (1998) *A summary of the colorectal cancer screening workshops and background papers.* London: NHS.

Oliver, S.E., May, M.T. and Gunnell, D. (2001) International trends in prostate-cancer mortality in the 'PSA ERA'. *International Journal of Cancer* 92, 893–898.

OXCHECK Study Group (1995) Effectiveness of health checks conducted by nurses in primary care: final results of the OXCHECK study. Imperial Cancer Research Fund OXCHECK Study Group. *British Medical Journal* 310, 1099–1104.

Pinsky, P.F. (2004) Results of a randomized controlled trail of prostate cancer screening. *Prostate.* 61, 371.

Quinn, M., Babb, P., Jones, J. and Allen, E. (1999) Effect of screening on incidence of and mortality from cancer of cervix in England: evaluation based on routinely collected statistics. *British Medical Journal* 318, 904–908.

Raffle, A.E. (2000) Honesty about new screening programmes is best policy. *British Medical Journal* 320, 872.

Sasieni, P. and Adams, J. (1999) Effect of screening on cervical cancer mortality in England and Wales: analysis of trends with an age period cohort model. *British Medical Journal* 318, 1244–1245.

Sasieni, P., Cuzick, J. and Farmery, E. (1995) Accelerated decline in cervical cancer mortality in England and Wales. *Lancet* 346, 1566–1567.

Schilling, F.H., Spix, C., Berthold, F., *et al.* (2002) Neuroblastoma screening at one year of age. *New England Journal of Medicine* 346, 1047–1053.

Shapiro, S. (1977) Evidence on screening for breast cancer from a randomized trial. *Cancer* 39, 6 Suppl., 2772–2782.

Sigurdsson, K., Adalsteinsson, S., Tulinius, H. and Ragnarsson, J. (1989) The value of screening as an approach to cervical cancer control in Iceland, 1964–1986. *International Journal of Cancer* 43, 1–5.

Thomas, D.B., Gao, D.L., Ray, R.M., *et al.* (2002) Randomized trial of breast self-examination in Shanghai: final results. *Journal of the National Cancer Institute* 94, 1445–1457.

Tsubono, Y. and Hisamichi, S. (2004) A halt to neuroblastoma screening in Japan. *New England Journal of Medicine* 350, 2010–2011.

UK Collaborative Trial of Ovarian Cancer Screening website. www.ukctocs.org.uk 0[accessed 16 November 2006].

UK Colorectal Cancer Screening Pilot Group (2004) Results of the first round of a demonstration pilot of screening for colorectal cancer in the United Kingdom. *British Medical Journal* 329, 133.

UKTEDBC (1988) First results on mortality reduction in the UK Trial of Early Detection of Breast Cancer. UK Trial of Early Detection of Breast Cancer Group. *Lancet* 2, 411–416.

US Department of Health and Human Services, Maternal and Child Health Bureau (2005) Newborn screening: toward a uniform screening panel and system—report for public comment. www.mchb.hrsa.gov/screening [accessed November 2006].

Welch, H.G. (2004) *Should I be tested for cancer? Maybe not and here's why.* Los Angeles: University of California Press.

Willis, B.H., Barton, P., Pearmain, P. and Bryan, S. (2005) Cervical screening programmes:can automation help? Evidence from systematic reviews, an economic analysis and a simulation modelling exercise applied to the UK. *Health Technology Assessment.* 9, 13 NHS RandD.

Winawer, S.J., Fletcher, R.H., Miller, L., *et al.* (1997) Colorectal cancer screening: clinical guidelines and rationale. *Gastroenterology* 112, 594–642.

Woods, W.G., Gao, R.N., Shuster, J., *et al.* (2002) Screening of infants and mortality due to neuroblastoma. *New England Journal of Medicine* 346, 1041–1046.

Chapter 5

Brown, M.L., Kessler, L.G. and Rueter, F.G. (1990) Is the supply of mammography machines outstripping need and demand? An economic analysis. *Annals of Internal Medicine* 113, 547–552.

Forrest, A.P.M. (1986) *Breast cancer screening.* Report to the health ministers for England, Wales, Scotland and Northern Ireland by a Working Group chaired by Sir Patrick Forrest. London: HMSO.

NHS Breast Screening Programme (2005) *Consolidated standards for the NHS breast screening programme.* Publication No 60 (version 2). Sheffield: NHS Cancer Screening Programmes.

NHS Cancer Screening Programmes Website. www.cancerscreening.nhs.uk [accessed June 2006].

O'Connor, A.M., Stacey, D., Rovner, D., *et al.* (2001) Decision aids for people facing health treatment or screening decisions. *Cochrane Database Systematic Review* no. 3, p. CD001431.

Chapter 6

Donabedian, A. (1996) Evaluating the quality of medical care. *Millbank Memorial Fund Quarterly* 44, 166–203.

Donabedian, A. (2003) *An introduction to quality assurance in health care.* Oxford: Oxford University Press.

Halberstam, D. (1986) *The reckoning*. New York: William Morrow and Co.

Ishikawa, K. (1985) *What is total quality control? The Japanese way*. Englewood Cliffs, NJ: Prentice Hall.

Mackenzie, D.G., Wild, S.H. and Rutledge, P. (2006) Are eligibility criteria for over the counter statins appropriate? *British Medical Journal* 333, 704.

Moynihan, R. and Cassels, A. (2005) *Selling sickness. How drug companies are turning us all into patients*. Crows Nest NSW Australia: Allen and Unwin.

NHS Cervical Screening programme (2003) *Modernising the NHS cervical screening programme; advice to the service. Annex B Frequency of cervical screening*. Sheffield: NHS Cancer Screening Programmes.

NHS National Library for Health Screening Specialist Sublibrary www.library.nhs.uk/screening/ [accessed July 2006].

NHS Sickle Cell and Thalassaemia Programme. Standards for the linked Antenatal and Newborn Screening Programme. www.kcl-phs.org.uk/haemscreening/Documents/ProgrammeSTAN.pdf [accessed 12 December 2006].

Surowiecki, J. (2005) *The wisdom of crowds. Why the many are smarter than the few*. London: Abacus.

Wilkinson, C.E., Peters, T.J., Harvey, I.M. and Stott, N.C. (1992) Risk targeting in cervical screening: a new look at an old problem. *British Journal of General Practice* 42, 435–438.

Chapter 7

Angell, M. (1990) *Science on trial. The clash of medical evidence and the law in the breast implant case*. New York: W.W. Norton and Co.

Austin, R.M. (1997) Results of blinded rescreening of Papanicolaou smears versus biased retrospective review. *Archives of Pathology and Laboratory Medicine* 121, 311–314.

Bell, R., Petticrew, M., Luengo, S. and Sheldon, T.A. (1998) Screening for ovarian cancer: a systematic review. *Health Technology Assessment* 2, 1–84.

British Medical Association Board of Science (2005) *Population screening and genetic testing. A briefing on current programmes and technologies*. London: British Medical Association.

DeMay, R.M. (1996) To err is human—to sue, American. *Diagnostic Cytopathology*, 15(3)iii–vi.

Frankel, S., Smith, G.D., Donovan, J. and Neal, D. (2003) Screening for prostate cancer. *Lancet* 361, 1122–1128.

General Medical Council (2006) *Management for doctors*. London: General Medical Council.

Jacobs, I.J., Skates, S.J., MacDonald, N., *et al.* (1999) Screening for ovarian cancer: a pilot randomised controlled trial. *Lancet* 353, 1207–1210.

Laitner, S. (2002) *Renal disease. Population screening for bladder cancer and glomerulonephritis, a review of the evidence with policy recommendations.* UK National Screening Committee.

Merenstein, D. (2004) A piece of my mind. Winners and losers. *Journal of the American Medical Association* 291, 15–16.

National Audit Office (1998) *Performance of the NHS Cervical Screening Programme in England.* London: HMSO.

Peticolas, A. (2003) Conductors on a one-way track: do medical authorities really get to decide policy about medical screening tests? *Medscape General Medicine* 5, 5.

Schwartz, L.M., Woloshin, S., Fowler, F.J., Jr and Welch, H.G. (2004) Enthusiasm for cancer screening in the United States. *Journal of the American Medical Association* 291, 71–78.

UK Collaborative Trial of Ovarian Cancer Screening website. www.ukctocs.org.uk [accessed 16 November 2006].

US Food and Drug Administration (2005) Whole body CT www.fda.gov/cdrh/ct [accessed June 2005].

Wells, W. (1997) *Review of cervical screening services at Kent and Canterbury Hospitals NHS Trust.* London: NHS Executive South Thames.

Which? (2004) *Health screens fail our tests.* August pp. 10–12

Chapter 8

Anonymous (1995) When is genetic screening permissible? *Nature* 377, 273.

Barnett, A. (2004) Revealed: how stars were hijacked to boost health company profits. *The Observer* Sunday 25 January.

Botkin, J.R., Clayton, E.W., Fost, N.C., *et al.* (2006) Newborn screening technology: proceed with caution. *Pediatrics* 117, 1793–1799.

Chamberlain, J., Melia, J., Moss, S. and Brown, J. (1997) The diagnosis, management, treatment and costs of prostate cancer in England and Wales. *Health Technology Assessment* 1, (3) pp. 1–53.

Chapman, S. (2006) Influencing governments via media advocacy. In: Pencheon, D., Guest C, Melzer, D. and Gray, M., ed. *Oxford handbook of public health practice,* 2nd edn. Oxford: Oxford University Press, pp. 348–353.

Coulter, A., ed. (2001) Informed choice in screening. *Health Expectations* 4, 79–139

Cross, T. (2002) *Prostate cancer screening in the UK: what factors are driving its implementation? A report for the national screening committee.* Health Policy Report. London: London School of Hygiene and Tropical Medicine.

Daniels, N. and Sabin, J. (1997) Limits to health care: fair procedures, democratic deliberation, and the legitimacy problem for insurers. *Philosophy and Public Affairs* 26, 303–350.

Daniels, N. and Sabin, J. (1998) The ethics of accountability in managed care reform. *Health Affairs (Millwood)* 17, 50–64.

Donovan, J.L., Frankel, S.J., Neal, D.E. and Hamdy, F.C. (2001) Screening for prostate cancer in the UK. Seems to be creeping in by the back door. *British Medical Journal* 323, 763–764.

Eddy, D.M. (1990) Screening for cervical cancer. *Annals of Internal Medicne* 113, 214–226.

Elwyn, G., O'Connor, A., Stacey, D., *et al.* (2006) Developing a quality criteria framework for patient decision aids: online international Delphi consensus process. *British Medical Journal* 333, 417.

Fahey, T., Griffiths, S. and Peters, T.J. (1995) Evidence based purchasing: understanding results of clinical trials and systematic reviews. *British Medical Journal* 311, 1056–1059.

Fletcher, S.W. (1997) Whither scientific deliberation in health policy recommendations? Alice in the Wonderland of breast-cancer screening. *New England Journal of Medicine* 336, 1180–1183.

Forrest, A.P.M. (1986) *Breast cancer screening.* Report to the health ministers for England, Wales, Scotland and Northern Ireland by a Working Group chaired by Sir Patrick Forrest. London: HMSO.

General Medical Council (1998) *Seeking patients' consent: the ethical considerations.* London: General Medical Council.

Gigerenzer, G. (2002) *Reckoning with risk.* London: Penguin.

Hardcastle, J.D., Chamberlain, J.O., Robinson, M.H., *et al.* (1996) Randomised controlled trial of faecal-occult-blood screening for colorectal cancer. *Lancet* 348, 1472–1477.

Harling, C., Gjini, A., Ruth, K. and Verne, J. (2005) *Trends in prostate cancer and its management in the South West Region, Hampshire and the Isle of Wight.* South West Public Health Observatory.

IARC Working Group. (1986) Screening for squamous cervical cancer: duration of low risk after negative results of cervical cytology and its implication for screening policies. IARC Working Group on evaluation of cervical cancer screening programmes. *British Medical Journal* 293, 659–664.

Knox, E.G. (1991) Case–control studies of screening procedures. *Public Health* 105, 55–61.

Law, M. (2004) Screening without evidence of efficacy. *British Medical Journal* 328, 7435, 301–302.

Levi, F., Lucchini, F., Negri, E., Franceschi, S. and la Vecchia, C. (2000) Cervical cancer mortality in young women in Europe: patterns and trends. *European Journal of Cancer* 36, 2266–2271.

Linos, A. and Riza, E. (2000) Comparisons of cervical cancer screening programmes in the European Union. *European Journal of Cancer* 36, 2260–2265.

Maissi, E., Marteau, T. M., Hankins, M., Moss, S., Legood, R. and Gray, A. (2004) Psychological impact of human papillomavirus testing in women with borderline or mildly dyskaryotic cervical smear test results: cross sectional questionnaire study. *British Medical Journal* 328, 1293.

Mayer, M. (2005) When clinical trials are compromised: a perspective from a patient advocate. *PLoS Med* 2, e358.

Moynihan, R. and Cassels, A. (2005) *Selling Sickness, how drug companies are turning us all into patients*. Crows Nest NSW Australia: Allen and Unwin.

Murphy, S.B., Cohn, S.L., Craft, A.W., *et al.* (1991) Do children benefit from mass screening for neuroblastoma? Consensus Statement from the American Cancer Society Workshop on Neuroblastoma Screening. *Lancet* 337, 344–346.

National Screening Committee (2003) *Criteria for appraising the viability, effectiveness and appropriateness of a screening programme*. UK National Screening Committee.

NHS Cancer Screening Programmes. Cervical screening, the facts. www.cancerscreening.nhs.uk [accessed June 2006] Sheffield.

NHS Cancer Screening Programmes. Prostate cancer risk management. http://www.cancerscreening.nhs.uk/prostate/pcrm-aim.html [accessed 28 November 2006].

NIH Consensus Development Panel (1997) National Institutes of Health Consensus Development Conference Statement: breast cancer screening for women ages 40–49, January 21–23, 1997. National Institutes of Health Consensus Developmental Panel. *Journal of the National Cancer Institute Monograph* no. 22, vii–xviii.

NIH National Cancer Advisory Board (1997) *National Cancer Advisory Board mammography recommendations for women ages 40 to 49*. Bethesda, MD: National Institutes of Health.

Oliver, S.E., Donovan, J.L., Peters, T.J., Frankel, S., Hamdy, F.C. and Neal, D.E. (2003) Recent trends in the use of radical prostatectomy in England: the epidemiology of diffusion. *BJU International* 91, 331–336.

Potosky, A.L., Legler, J., Albertsen, P.C., *et al.* (2000) Health outcomes after prostatectomy or radiotherapy for prostate cancer: results from the Prostate Cancer Outcomes Study. *Journal of the National Cancer Institute* 92, 1582–1592.

Quinn, M., Babb, P., Brock, A., Kirby, L. and Jones, J. (2001) *Cancer trends in England and Wales*. London: Office for National Statistics.

Raffle, A.E. (2006) Lasting damage from the trastuzumab storm. *British Medical Journal* 333,761.

Raffle, A.E. (1998) New tests in cervical screening. *Lancet* 351, 297.

Raffle, A.E., Alden, B., Quinn, M., Babb, P.J. and Brett, M.T. (2003) Outcomes of screening to prevent cancer: analysis of cumulative incidence of cervical abnormality and modelling of cases and deaths prevented. *British Medical Journal* 326, 901.

Rawls, J. (1971) *A theory of justice.* Cambridge, MA: Harvard University Press.

Roberts, M.M. (1989) Breast screening: time for a rethink? *British Medical Journal* 299, 1153–1155.

Russell, L.B. (1994) Eduated guesses; making policy about medical screening tests. London: University of California Press.

Sackett, D.L. and Holland, W.W. (1975) Controversy in the detection of disease. *Lancet* 2, 357–359.

Savulescu, J., Hendrick, J. and Hope, T. (2003) *Medical ethics and law; the core curriculum* Edinburgh: Churchill Livingstone.

Selley, S., Donovan, J., Faulkner, A., Coast, J. and Gillatt, D. (1997) Diagnosis, management and screening of early localised prostate cancer. *Health Technology Assessment* 1, (2) pp. 1–96.

Skrabanek, P. (1994) *The death of humane medicine.* London: Social Affairs Unit.

Soutter, W.P., de Barros, L.A., Fletcher, A., Monaghan, J.M., Duncan, I.D., Paraskevaidis, E. and Kitchener, H.C. (1997) Invasive cervical cancer after conservative therapy for cervical intraepithelial neoplasia. *Lancet* 349, 978–980.

Stamey, T.A., Caldwell, M., McNeal, J.E., Nolley, R., Hemenez, M. and Downs, J. (2004) The prostate specific antigen era in the United States is over for prostate cancer: what happened in the last 20 years? *Journal of Urology* 172, 1297–1301.

Towler, B.P., Irwig, L., Glasziou, P., Weller, D. and Kewenter, J. (2000) Screening for colorectal cancer using the faecal occult blood test, hemoccult. *Cochrane Database Systematic Review* no. 2, p. CD001216.

Tsubono, Y. and Hisamichi, S. (2004) A halt to neuroblastoma screening in Japan. *New England Journal of Medicine* 350, 2010–2011.

UK clinical ethics network (2004) Resource allocation in health care. www.ethics-network.org.uk/Ethics/eresource.htm [accessed 25 November 2006].

UK National Screening Committee (2000) *Second report of the UK National Screening Committee.* Departments of Health for England, Scotland, Northern Ireland and Wales.

University of Bristol. ProtecT Study website (Prostate testing for cancer and Treatment). www.epi.bris.ac.uk/protect [accessed 28 November 2006].

van Ballegooijen, M., van den Akker-van Marle, Patnick, J., *et al.* (2000) Overview of important cervical cancer screening process values in European Union (EU) countries, and tentative predictions of the corresponding effectiveness and cost-effectiveness. *European Journal of Cancer* 36, 2177–2188.

Watson, R. (2001) European women's group calls for human papillomavirus testing. *British Medical Journal* 323, 772.

Weatherall, D.J. (2000) Single gene disorders or complex traits: lessons from the thalassaemias and other monogenic diseases. *British Medical Journal* 321, 1117–1120.

Wilkinson, C.E., Peters, T.J., Harvey, I.M. and Stott, N.C. (1992) Risk targeting in cervical screening: a new look at an old problem. *British Journal of General Practice* 42, 435–438.

Williams, A. (1985) Economics of coronary artery bypass grafting. *British Medical Journal* 291, 326–329.

Woodman, C.B., Collins, S., Winter, H., *et al.* (2001) Natural history of cervical human papillomavirus infection in young women: a longitudinal cohort study. *Lancet* 357, 1831–1836.

Index